Alexander Monro

Three treatises: on the brain, the eye and the ear

Alexander Monro

Three treatises: on the brain, the eye and the ear

ISBN/EAN: 9783741104015

Manufactured in Europe, USA, Canada, Australia, Japa

Cover: Foto ©Lupo / pixelio.de

Manufactured and distributed by brebook publishing software
(www.brebook.com)

Alexander Monro

Three treatises: on the brain, the eye and the ear

THREE TREATISES.

ON

THE BRAIN, THE EYE, AND THE EAR.

ILLUSTRATED BY TABLES.

BY

ALEXANDER MONRO, M. D.

PROFESSOR OF MEDICINE, ANATOMY, AND SURGERY, IN THE UNIVERSITY OF EDINBURGH; FELLOW OF THE ROYAL COLLEGE OF PHYSICIANS, AND OF THE ROYAL SOCIETY, OF EDINBURGH; AND FELLOW OF THE ROYAL ACADEMY OF SURGERY OF PARIS.

EDINBURGH:
PRINTED FOR BELL & BRADFUTE;
AND FOR G. G. & J. ROBINSON, AND J. JOHNSON,
LONDON.

M.DCC.XCVII.

OBSERVATIONS

ON THE

COMMUNICATION

OF THE

VENTRICLES OF THE BRAIN

WITH EACH OTHER;

AND ON THE

INTERNAL HYDROCEPHALUS.

BY

ALEXANDER MONRO, M. D.

PROFESSOR OF MEDICINE, ANATOMY, AND SURGERY,

IN THE UNIVERSITY OF EDINBURGH.

EDINBURGH:

PRINTED BY ADAM NEILL AND COMPANY.

1797.

GENERAL

TABLE OF CONTENTS.

A Table of the Contents of Treatiſe I.

CHAP. I.

CHAP. II.

CHAP. III.

CHAP. IV.

CHAP.

TREATISE

TREATISE FIRST:

OF THE BRAIN.

CHAP. I.

Of the Communication of the Ventricles of the Brain with each other, in Man and Quadrupeds.

SO far back as the year 1753, ſoon after I began the ſtudy of Anatomy, I diſcovered, that the Lateral Ventricles of the Human Brain communicated with each other, and, at the ſame place, with the Middle or Third Ventricle of the Brain: And, as a paſſage from the Third Ventricle to the Fourth is univerſally known, it followed, that what are called the Four Ventricles of the Brain, are in reality different parts of one cavity.

In confirmation of this, I afterwards obſerved, in the bodies of fifteen different perſons who had died of Internal Hydrocephalus, that the water was lodged in all the Ventricles; that by one puncture it was diſcharged from all of them; and that the paſſages by which I had found the Ventricles communicated, were dilated in the ſame proportion as the other parts of the Ventricles.

If, therefore, there has been no miſtake in the obſervations of thoſe who tell us, that in Hydrocephalus they have found the water confined to One of the Lateral Ventricles, or diſcharged by a puncture from One Ventricle, without emptying the others; there muſt have been, previous to the Dropſy, ſome degree of inflammation, or other diſeaſe, in that part of the brain, which had occaſioned an obliteration of their natural communications.

I found likewiſe, that there is no paſſage, ſuch as Dr Haller, and other authors, ſuppoſed, (See Haller, El. Phyſ. L. x. S. 2. § 6. p. 77. and S. 3. § 7. p. 87.) leading from the Cavity of the Fourth Ventricle into the Cavity, as it is called, of the Spinal Marrow, or, between the Dura and Pia Mater of the Spinal Marrow.

In

In the year 1764, I read a paper on that ſubject to the Philoſophical Society of Edinburgh: And, in 1783, when I publiſhed my book upon the Nervous Syſtem, I gave ſuch a full deſcription of the Communications of the Ventricles of the Brain, illuſtrated by figures, that I did not ſuppoſe any perſon, who pretended to anatomical knowledge, could find difficulty in tracing by diſſection all I had deſcribed.

To my very great ſurpriſe, however, I have been informed, that ſeveral Teachers of Anatomy in London have told their Pupils, that they had looked for ſuch paſſages in vain; and therefore ventured to deny their exiſtence.

But I cannot admit their inference: becauſe, in the firſt place, I have found, on repeating my diſſections in private, that the deſcriptions I publiſhed in 1783 are ſo correct, that I obſerve nothing material to add to, or to alter in them.

In the next place, ſince I heard of thoſe doubts as to the facts I had deſcribed, I have demonſtrated, annually, to all the Students of Anatomy who have done me the honour of attending my Lectures, every thing I had mentioned. Particularly, laſt winter, after I had demonſtrated theſe parts in one ſubject, I diſſected another, of which my aſſiſtant Mr

Fyfe made a very accurate drawing; which I ſhewed to all the Students, who compared it with the ſubject.

But, that no doubt might remain with the moſt ſceptical perſon, I have, this ſummer, repeated the diſſection of a recent ſubject; of which, likewiſe, Mr Fyfe made a very accurate drawing, that correſponds exactly with his former figure.

I then aſked the favour of all my Colleagues of the Medical Faculty, to wit, Dr Black, Dr Home, Dr Rutherford, Dr Gregory, and Dr Duncan, to compare the Drawings with the parts diſſected; which they were ſo obliging as to do: And I ſubjoin their Declaration.

After they had finiſhed their compariſon of the Drawing marked Table Firſt, with the diſſected Brain; I held the end of a blow-pipe at the diſtance of half an inch from the hole by which the Lateral Ventricles communicate; and, on my blowing moderately, I ſhewed them, that the air paſſed from the Right into the Left Lateral Ventricle.

I then opened the Left Lateral Ventricle, and pointed out to them the hole by which the air had paſſed.

I

I afterwards made a Caſt in Paris Plaſter of the Parts repreſented in the Firſt Figure: And this caſt, which I preſerve, correſponds exactly with the Drawing and Engraving.

DECLARATION by the PROFESSORS of the FACULTY of PHYSIC in the Univerſity of Edinburgh.

" WE whoſe names are ſubſcribed hereby declare, That on " the 13th day of June 1794, Dr MONRO demonſtrated to " us, in the Anatomical Theatre, the Human Brain cut per- " pendicularly at the right ſide of its Septum Lucidum; and, " along with it, a Drawing of it, marked Table Firſt, juſt " finiſhed by Mr FYFE: That we examined and compared " theſe accurately together, and found them to correſpond " in all reſpects; particularly, we ſaw diſtinctly a hole or " paſſage by which the Lateral Ventricles communicate with " each other, and with the Third Ventricle.

" After this, Dr MONRO placed the ſmall end of a com-
" mon blow-pipe about half an inch from this hole or paſ-
" ſage ; and, on his blowing air gently, we ſaw it paſs
" through the above-mentioned hole or paſſage into the Left
" Lateral Ventricle.

" He afterwards ſhewed us the Left Lateral Ventricle
" laid open, and a Drawing of its parts by Mr FYFE,
" marked Table Second ; and particularly, we ſaw the left
" ſide of the paſſage which makes the communication be-
" tween the Ventricles.

" He has, ſince that time, ſhewed us a Caſt in Paris
" Plaſter of the Parts repreſented in Table Firſt, which we
" find to correſpond exactly with the Drawing and Engra-
" ving.

" We therefore entertain no doubt of the exiſtence of the
" Communication of the Lateral Ventricles of the Brain
" with each other, and with the Third Ventricle, deſcribed
" by Dr MONRO in the Work he publiſhed on the Nervous
" Syſtem in 1783 ; and particularly, we atteſt the accuracy
" of the Figures and Deſcription of theſe Parts which he
" ſhewed

" ſhewed us, and which he propoſes to preſent to the Royal " Society of Edinburgh for publication.

" JOSEPH BLACK.

" FRANCIS HOME.

" JAMES GREGORY.

" D. RUTHERFORD.

" ANDREW DUNCAN."

MY very ingenious and intelligent Colleague Dr RUTHERFORD, who, as one of the ordinary Phyſicians of the Royal Infirmary, as well as one of the Clinical Lecturers there, has had frequent opportunity of examining this ſubject, has very obligingly favoured me with his farther atteſtation concerning it in the following Letter.

" For

" For Dr MONRO.

" Dear Sir,

" I am very much pleaſed with your Drawings and De-
" ſcription of the Communication of the Lateral Ventricles
" with each other, and with the other Ventricles of the
" Brain. The Firſt Figure is particularly excellent; and
" muſt certainly, I ſhould think, remove all doubts reſpecting
" the reality of theſe paſſages. It ſeems indeed very ſtrange,
" that ſo many celebrated Anatomiſts ſhould have miſſed the
" Communication betwixt the Lateral Ventricles; as it is ſo
" eaſily diſcovered, and as it is generally ſo very conſpicuous
" when the Ventricles are diſtended by water preternaturally
" accumulated in them. Frequently, when examining the
" ſtate of the Brain in perſons who had died in the Royal In-
" firmary, I have taken the opportunity of pointing out this
" Communication to the Young Gentlemen who were preſent
" at the diſſection; and have ſatisfied ſome, that it was al-
" ways to be found, who had been taught that no ſuch Com-
" munication exiſted. I particularly recollect one inſtance
" of this. A very ingenious and well-informed American,
" Mr

" Mr Philip Physick, who got his degree of M. D. at our
" Univerſity two years ago, and who had previouſly ap-
" plied cloſely to the ſtudy of Anatomy, and made great
" proficiency in it, under ſome of the moſt eminent Teach-
" ers in London, requeſted me to ſhew him the Communica-
" tion betwixt the Lateral Ventricles, as he had never been
" able to perceive it. I did ſo; and he viewed it then, for
" the firſt time, with much ſurpriſe. It is not poſſible to miſ-
" take it for an accidental laceration, the edge is ſo ex-
" tremely neat, ſmooth and regular. No doubt, it is more
" diſtinct in ſome inſtances than in others; and it may be,
" that, if the Ventricles were only juſt moiſt or without any
" ſenſible quantity of liquid collected in them, the ſurfaces
" conſequently quite contiguous to each other, it ſhould not
" be very apparent, and might therefore be overlooked by
" one prepoſſeſſed with the idea that no natural communica-
" tion did there exiſt. But I have never ſeen the Brain in
" ſuch ſtate, but that it was very eaſy to perceive it. When
" water is preternaturally collected in the Lateral Ventricles,
" it is ſometimes obſerved to be contained in much greater
" quantity in one of them, than in the other; and I have
" ſeen one of the Ventricles much enlarged and full of water,
" while the other remained of its natural capacity and con-
" tained hardly any water. This appearance I ſhould, how-

" ever, impute, not to the obliteration or obſtruction of the " communication betwixt them; but to one ſide of the Brain " having been more affected with diſeaſe, more flaccid and " tender, than the other; in conſequence of which, a greater " exſudation had taken place from the veſſels of this part, " and the ſides of the Ventricle had yielded more readily to " the preſſure of the water as it was effuſed.

" I remain, with much reſpect and eſteem,

" Dear Sir,

" Your moſt obedient humble ſervant,

EDINBURGH, 14*th Auguſt* 1794.

" D. RUTHERFORD."

As the Human Anatomy is generally illuſtrated by a Compariſon with other Animals, I next diſſected the Brain of the Ox and of the Sheep, in the ſame manner; of which Mr. FYFE drew accurate Figures. Theſe were compared with the Diſſected Brains by three of my Colleagues, to wit, Dr GRE-

GORY,

GORY, Dr RUTHERFORD, and Dr DUNCAN ; who allow me to add, that they were equally ſatisfied with the Accuracy of theſe Figures.

I found, that in theſe Animals, (and I have ſince obſerved the ſame in the Horſe and in the Whale), the middle parts of the Thalami Nervorum Opticorum are incorporated intimately, and hence, from the Paſſage by which the Lateral Ventricles communicate with each other and with the Third Ventricle, there is a Paſſage above, as well as below, the joining of the Thalami.

As this joining, and all other circumſtances of the ſtructure, are ſo nearly the ſame in the Ox, the Horſe, and the Sheep, I think it ſufficient to publiſh the Figure taken from the Ox.

EXPLANATION

OF THE

T A B L E S.

IN the defcription I am about to give of thefe Tables, I fhall place the Letters to which I refer, on an Outline of the Tables.

Explanation of Table Firft.

THIS Table reprefents the Human Cranium and Encephalon, cut perpendicularly at the right fide of the Falx and Septum Lucidum.

A A Reprefents the Section of the Cranium.

B A Section of the Right Frontal Sinus.

C

TAB. I.

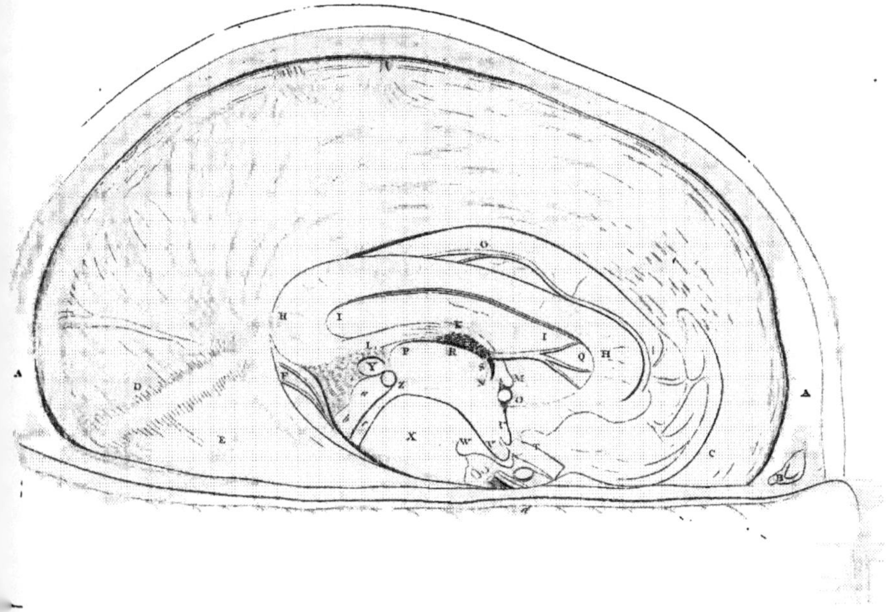

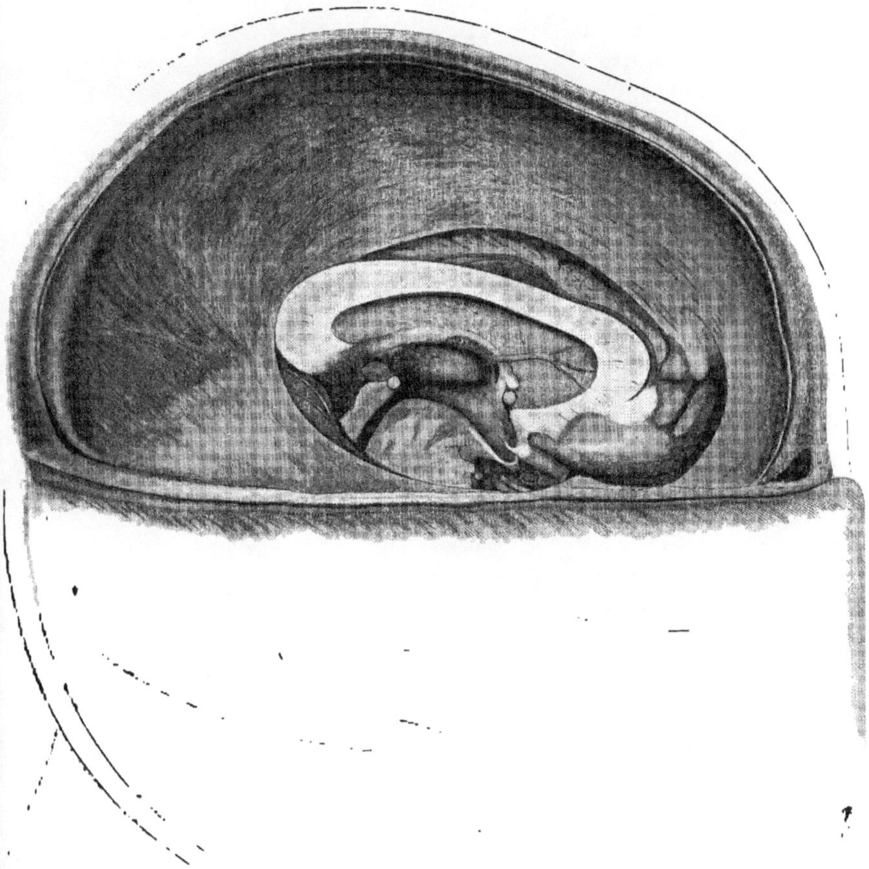

C The Forepart of the Falx, fixed to the Criſta Galli.

D The Backpart of the Falx, fixed to the Middle of the Tentorium, E.

F The Upper and Anterior Part of the Cerebellum.

G Part of the Inner-ſide of the Left Hemiſphere of the Brain, with Arteries upon its ſurface from the Anterior Branch of the Internal Carotid Artery.

H H A Section of the Corpus Calloſum.

I I The Septum Lucidum, between the Lateral Ventricles, in which there is no Hole.

K The Middle Part, or Body, of the Fornix.

L A Section of the Right Poſterior Crus of the Fornix.

M A Section of the Right Anterior Crus of the Fornix.

N The Left Anterior Crus of the Fornix.

O A Section of the Anterior Commiſſura Cerebri.

P The Inner-ſide of the Left Thalamus Nervi Optici, forming the Left Side of the Third Ventricle.

Q A Vein running on the Right Side of the Forepart of the Septum Lucidum, and then acroſs the Forepart of the Body of the Fornix, to terminate in the Choroid Plexus, R, under the Body of the Fornix, to which the Choroid Plexuſes of the two Lateral Ventricles are united.

S An Oval Hole, ſituated under the Anterior Part of the Body of the Fornix; behind the Anterior Crura of the Fornix and Commiſſura Anterior Cerebri; on the Forepart of the Joining of the Choroid Plexuſes of the two Lateral Ventricles of the Brain; and over the Forepart of the Third Ventricle. Hence, at at this place, the Lateral Ventricles of the Brain communicate with each other and with the Third Ventricle.

T The Left Optic Nerve cut away from the Right at the place of their Junction.

U A Blind Sac in the Left Side of the Third Ventricle; under the Commiſſura Anterior, and between the Continuation of the Corpus Calloſum and the Joining of the Left Optic Nerve with its Thalamus.

V The Iter per Infundibulum ad Glandulam Pituitariam, between the Joining of the Optic Nerves with their Thalami and the Corpora Albicantia; a Section of the Right one of which is repreſented at W.

X A Section of the Tuber Annulare.

Y The Pineal Gland, fixed by a Peduncle on each ſide to the Thalami Nervorum Opticorum, and by a middle Peduncle to Z, the Commiſſura Cerebri Poſterior.

a

a The Nates of the Right Side cut.

b The Teſtis of the Right Side cut.

c The Iter a Tertio ad Quartum Ventriculum.

d A Section of the Right Internal Carotid Artery.

Explanation

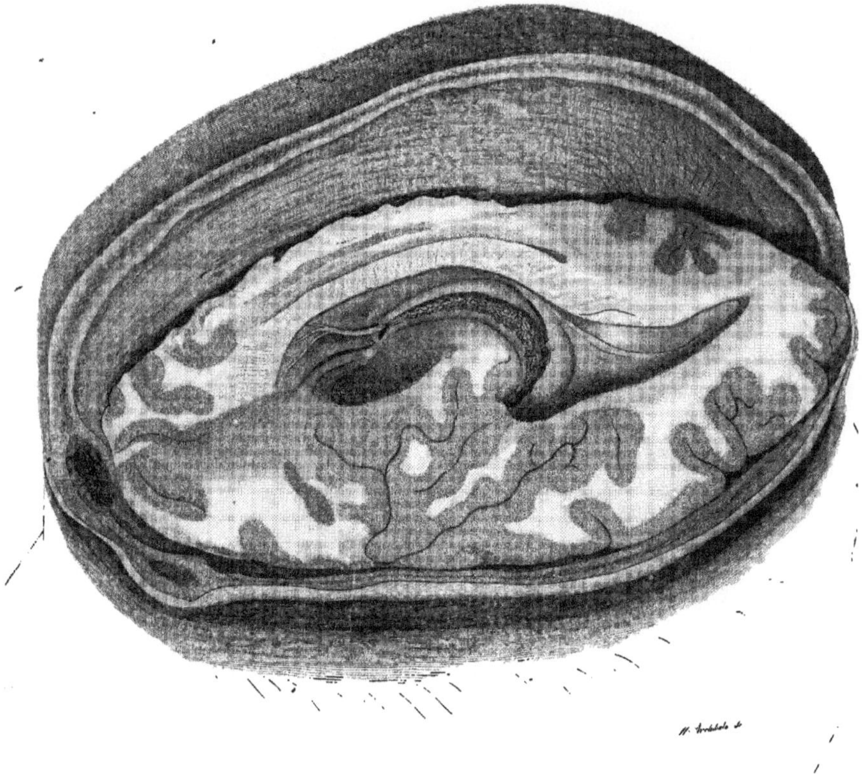

TAB. II

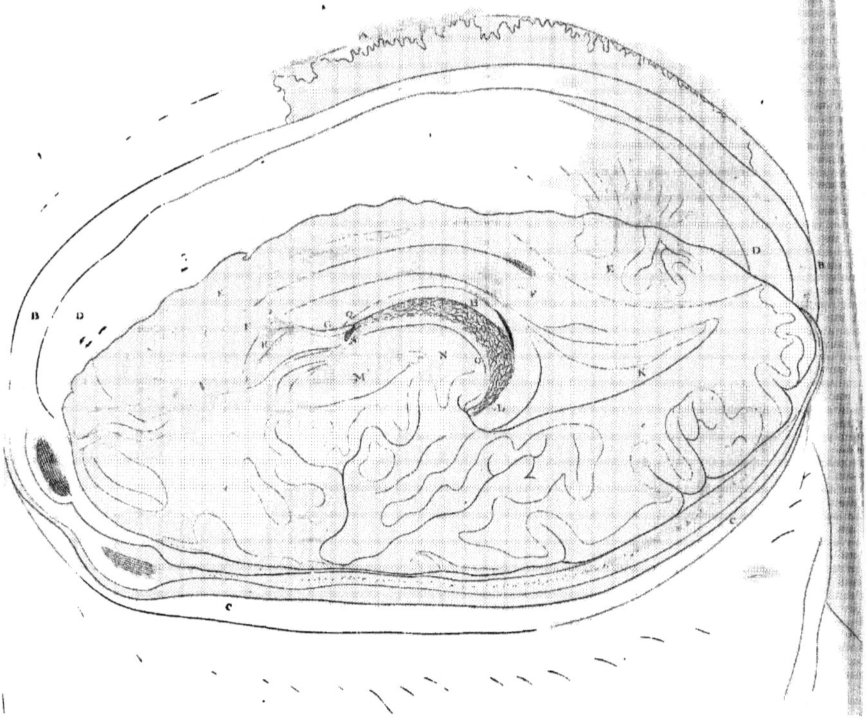

Explanation of Table Second.

THIS Table repreſents the Cranium and the Left Hemiſphere of the Brain of the ſame ſubject; cut, firſt, perpendicularly, about the diſtance of a finger-breadth from the Falx, to ſuch a depth as to lay open the Left Lateral Ventricle; and then cut, almoſt horizontally, from the Septum Lucidum and Left Ventricle, to the Outer-ſide of the Left Hemiſphere of the Brain.

A The Sagittal Suture of the Cranium.

B B The Cut Edge of the Top of the Cranium.

C C An Horizontal Section of the Cranium.

D D The Left Side of the Falx.

E E The Inner-part of the Left Hemiſphere, cut perpendicularly.

e e The Outer-part of the Left Hemiſphere, cut almoſt horizontally.

F F A perpendicular Section of the Corpus Calloſum.

G The Septum Lucidum.

H The Middle Part or Body of the Fornix.

I Part of the Anterior Cornu of the Lateral Ventricle.

K The Poſterior Cornu of the Lateral Ventricle.

L The Left Pes Hippocampi.

M A Section of the Left Corpus Striatum.

N

N A Section of the Left Thalamus Nervi Optici.

O The Choroid Plexus of the Left Ventricle.

R Veins running on the Forepart of the Septum Lucidum, which pass over Q, the Left Anterior Crus of the Fornix, to terminate where the Choroid Plexuses of the Two Ventricles are joined to the Choroid Plexus under the Body of the Fornix.

S The Left Side of the Oval Hole or Passage by which the Lateral Ventricles communicate with each other and with the Third Ventricle.

Explanation of Table Third.

THIS Table repreſents the Cranium and the Encephalon of an Ox, cut perpendicularly on the Right Side of the Falx Cerebri.

A A A Section of the Cranium.

B B The Falx, which is narrower in proportion to the Brain than it is in Man.

C The Inner-ſide of the Left Hemiſphere of the Brain.

D D A Section of the Corpus Calloſum.

F

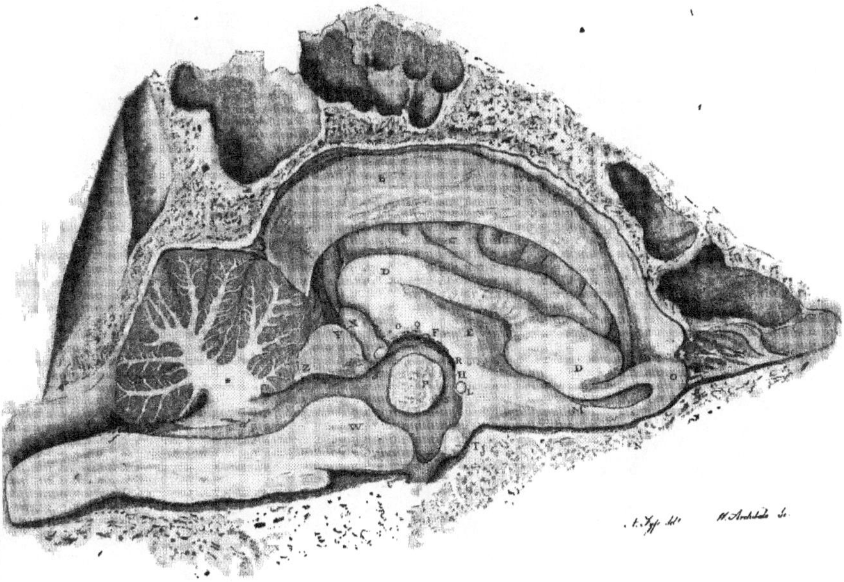
A. Fyfe del.
W. Archibald sc.

E The Septum Lucidum.

F The Middle Part, or Body, of the Fornix.

G The place from which its Right Poſterior Crus was cut off.

H A Section of its Right Anterior Crus.

L A Section of the Anterior Commiſſura Cerebri.

M A longitudinal Section of the Right Olfactory Nerve, from its Origin to the Ethmoid Bone.

N A Canal, or Tube, which begins in the Forepart of the Lateral Ventricle, and is continued obliquely downwards within the Optic Nerve, enlarging near to the End of the Nerve. The Inner-ſides of it are medullary; and the End of it, which is ſhut or blind, is covered with a cineritious Bulb, O; from which the Fibres of the Olfactory Nerve are derived.

P

P A thick Medullary Cord cut, by which the Thalami of the Optic Nerves are united.

Q The Choroid Plexus under the Body of the Fornix.

R An Oval Hole by which the Lateral Ventricles communicate with each other and with the Third Ventricle.

S A Paſſage leading downwards, between the Anterior Commiſſura Cerebri, and the Joining or Commiſſura of the Thalami Nervorum Opticorum.

T A Section of the Right Optic Nerve where it is joined to its Fellow.

U A Section of the Right Corpus Albicans.

V The Infundibulum, between the Joining of the Optic Nerves and the Corpora Albicantia.

W A Section of the Tuber Annulare.

X The Pineal Gland.

Y A Section of the Right Nates.

Z A Section of the Right Testis.

* A Section of the Cerebellum.

a A Section of the Commissura Cerebri Posterior.

b A Passage, from the Hole by which the Lateral Ventricles communicate with each other and with the Third Ventricle, leading to *c*, or to the Iter ad Quartum Ventriculum.

d The Cavity of the Fourth Ventricle.

e The Spinal Marrow, consisting of two principal Cords.

f

f The Bottom of the Fourth Ventricle, ſhut by its Choroid Plexus and Pia Mater; ſo that there is no Communication between the Cavity of the Fourth Ventricle and the Cavity of the Spinal Marrow.

CHAP.

TAB IV.

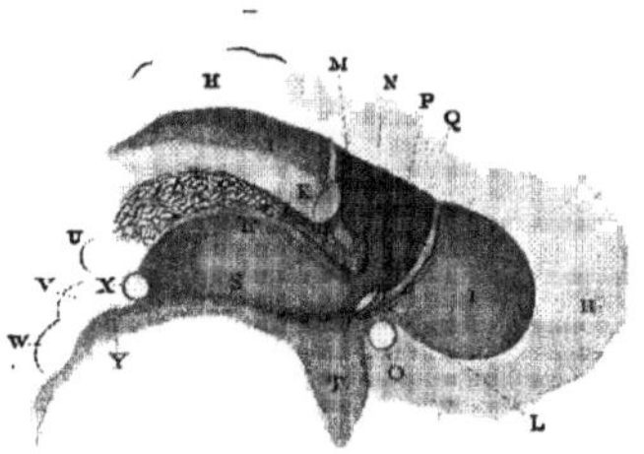

A Fyfe del. W. Archibald Sc.

Explanation of Table Fourth.

In this Table, the Septum Lucidum, and the Fornix, immediately behind its Anterior Crura, are cut acrofs, in order to fhew, ftill more fully, the Paffage by which the Lateral Ventricles of the Brain communicate with each other and with the Third Ventricle.

H H A Longitudinal Section of the Corpus Callofum, on the Right Side of the Septum Lucidum.

I I The Septum Lucidum.

K A Section of the Septum Lucidum, and of the Body of the Fornix, behind its Anterior Crura.

L The Right Anterior Crus of the Fornix.

M The Joining of the Choroid Plexufes of the Lateral Ventricles.

N A Part of the Left Tænia, or Left Centrum Semicirculare Geminum.

O The Section of the Commissura Cerebri Anterior.

P Part of the Cavity of the Left Lateral Ventricle.

Q The Bottom of the Passage by which the Lateral Ventricles communicate with each other and with the Third Ventricle.

R The Joining of the Thalami Nervorum Opticorum, cut.

S The Left Side of the Third Ventricle.

T The Passage downwards to the Infundibulum.

U The Outline of the Pineal Gland.

V W The Outline of the Right Natis and Testis, cut.

X The Section of the Commissura Cerebri Posterior.

Y The Iter ad Quartum Ventriculum.

CHAP.

CHAP. II.

Of the Situation of the Water in the Internal Hydrocephalus.

AN Anatomiſt, reaſoning *à priore*, would be apt to ſuppoſe, that the Water, in the Hydrocephalus Internus, ſhould be as often found immediately within the Dura Mater, between it and the Outer-ſide of the Brain, Cerebellum, and Spinal Marrow, as within the Ventricles of the Brain. Experience, however, proves that it is generally collected within the Ventricles; and, as I have not met with a ſingle inſtance in which the Water was entirely on the Outer-ſide of the Brain, (although I am far from doubting of the poſſibility of the fact), I cannot help ſuſpecting that this happens much more rarely than is ſuppoſed by Authors; and that in many caſes, ſuppoſed to have been of this kind, the

Brain had been lacerated in opening the Cranium, and the Water by that means effufed on the Surface of the Brain.

In many other cafes, where a great quantity of it was collected within the Head, although part of it was, during life, fituated on the Outer-fide of the Brain, and run out as foon as the Dura Mater was cut; it is certain that the Water had begun to collect within the Ventricles of the Brain, and had efcaped from them afterwards in confequence of Changes in the Solid Texture of the Brain, which I fhall endeavour to prove, in the next Chapter, frequently take place.

CHAP.

CHAP. III.

Of Changes produced in the Texture of the Brain and Cerebellum, in consequence of Hydrocephalus Internus.

THE disease named Internal Hydrocephalus, in which the Water is at first contained within the Ventricles of the Brain, has been divided by some Authors, not improperly, into two species; the *Acute*, and the *Chronic*.

In the Acute, the disease generally proves fatal in less than the space of a month; and it is seldom that more than two or three ounces of Water are found within the Ventricles. From the smallness of the quantity, no uncommon separation of the bones from each other, or opening of the futures, is diftinguifhable.

In the Chronic fpecies of the difeafe, the patient furvives for many months, fometimes for a year or two. The bones of the Cranium are feparated from each other; in fome cafes to a great diftance. In the foft fpaces between them, the undulation of a fluid is more or lefs diftinguifhable, according to the age of the patient and progrefs of the difeafe. In a few cafes, I have feen the bones feparated to a confiderable diftance from each other, although the difeafe did not begin till the child was upwards of two years of age.

In this fpecies, from two to five pounds of Water have often been found within the Cranium; and fometimes a much greater quantity *.

When

* See BONET. Sepulchr. L. i. S. 16. MORGAGNI, Ep. xii. LIEUTAUD, L. 3. S. 5. and others.

When one, two, or three pounds only of Water were collected, it has been generally confined within the Ventricles of the Brain; the ſides of which, or ſubſtance of the Brain bounding the Ventricles, were obſerved to be much thinner* than they are in health: And as the Bones at the top of the Cranium are more looſely connected than thoſe at its baſe, the Subſtance of the Brain which covers the Ventricles, or the upper part of its hemiſpheres, is in proportion more dilated than the under part of the Brain. In ſome inſtances, the Subſtance of the Brain appeared to be ſomewhat indurated; in others, it ſeemed to be ſoftened.

Where the quantity of Water amounted to five, ſix, or more pounds, partial Adheſions of the Surface of the Brain to the Dura Mater were obſerved; at the ſame time, a quantity run out on opening the Cranium and Dura Mater†.

On

* MORGAGNI, Ep. xii. 5. "Cerebrum Hydrocephalo attenuatum." 8. "Parietum "Lateralium Ventriculorum craſſitudo vi aquæ extenuata." LIEUTAUD, L. 3. Obſ. 322. "A mole aquæ, Cerebrum in ambitu ſemipollicis craſſitiem vix ſuper-"abat."

† MORGAGNI, Ep. xii. 6. "Aqua ad primam cultri impreſſionem, cum impetu "prorumpens."

On examining farther, the Cortical and Medullary Subſtances were found to be greatly diminiſhed in their bulk and weight. In ſome caſes, after an enormous Diſtenſion of the Ventricles of the Brain, large portions of the ſolid Subſtance of the Brain ſeemed to have been deſtroyed; and hence, the Water was partly lodged within the Ventricles, and partly between the Surface of the Brain and the Dura Mater *.

In other caſes, little remained of the Brain, except its inveſting membranes, with ſome of the ſuperficial matter adhering to them; and the oſſeous matter of ſome of the bones of the Cranium, was found to be likewiſe waſted †.

In

* In a caſe of a Child (C. Gilles, 18 months old,) which occurred in our Infirmary in 1778, five pounds of Water were found, partly within the Ventricles, and partly between the Dura Mater and Brain. The Subſtance of the Brain appeared ſoft and flabby; and its texture, in many parts, was much deſtroyed.

† Lieutaud, L. 3. Obſ. 326. Miſcel. Cur. Tredecem Aquæ libræ intra Ventriculos et totum Cerebrum nonniſi ſaccum referebat.—327. Ex Hildano Aquæ libræ

In a fœtus Calf, within a few days of the common time of parturition, I found the Cranium enormouſly dilated, and nearly of a ſpherical figure. On opening the Cranium and Dura Mater with great care, I found the Arachnoid Coat with the Pia Mater, both of the Brain and Cerebellum, in contact with the Dura Mater, and in ſome places adhering to it. On cutting theſe, I found thin and broken-like portions of cineritious-looking ſubſtance adhering to them; and, within this, upwards of fifteen pounds of a tranſparent watery liquor, a ſmall proportion only of which coagulated on boiling it. I afterwards cut out all the membranes of the Brain and Cerebellum, with the cineritious-looking matter adhering to them, and found that the whole weighed only one ounce and a half.

In

---

libræ octo: ipſummet Cerebrum in ſacculum extendebatur, Cranium paſſim membranoſum, potius quam oſſeum, videbatur.—328. Cerebrum in ſaccum extenſum.—329. Aquæ copia Cerebrum ferme obliterabat.—332. Ex KERKRING. Cerebri loco, Aqua.

MORGAGNI, Ep. xii. 5. Cerebrum Hydrocephalo attenuatum. — 8. Cerebrum prima inſpectione nullum eſſe videbatur, cum, inſtar craſſioris membranæ, adhæreſceret undique arcuatæ diſſolutorum oſſium circumferentiæ. — 8. Radicem Cerebri in fibras diffluxiſſe.

In Sheep labouring under the diſeaſe commonly called the Staggers, I have found a Bag, containing a watery fluid, and bodies which have been ſuppoſed to be animated, (and which I have no doubt are ſo), in one of the hemiſpheres of the Brain. Over the Bag, the bottom of which was connected to the bottom of one of the Lateral Ventricles, I found the Medullary and Cineritious Subſtances of the Brain conſumed, and the Bag adhering to the Pia Mater, and the Pia Mater with the Arachnoid Coat adhering to the Dura Mater; and over that part of the Dura Mater, the oſſeous ſubſtance of the Cranium was wanting, and a membrane ſeemed to ſupply its place. On inquiry, I find, that Sheep-graziers diſtinguiſh with certainty the ſituation of this diſeaſe, by feeling a ſoft place in the Cranium, at which they make a perforation, and endeavour to extract the Sac or Bag; but, as the ſubſtance of the Brain is deeply affected by the diſeaſe, few are ſaved by the operation.

CHAP. IV.

An Attempt to prove, that the Changes in the Texture of the Brain and Cerebellum, in consequence of Internal Hydrocephalus, are produced by the Absorbent Vessels.

IT has been, so far as I know, the universal opinion of Anatomists and Physicians, that, in the Hydrocephalus Internus, the Substance of the Brain is melted down by the Watery Liquor which is effused from the Arteries.

To ſhew that they have thought ſo, I ſhall, at the foot of the page, ſubjoin a few quotations from ſome of the moſt eminent Authors *.

As

* Boneti, Sep. L. i. S. 16. Obſ. 11. " Nam potuit Cerebrum per redundans " ſerum adeo fuiſſe emollitum ut mucus eſſe viſum fuerit." S. 16. Ad. Obſ. 5. " Radix Cerebri, a perpetuo illo diluvio et ſeri incubitu, in fibras diffluxiſſe vide- " batur."

Morgagni, de Sed. et Cur. Morb. Ep. xii. 5. " Cerebrum in Hydrocephalo at- " tenuatum et in aquam reſolutum."—6. " Quod ſi Cerebrum ſit Hydrocephali " aqua diſſolutum."—6. Verum quacunque ratione et quocunque ex fonte intra Ce- " rebri thecam aqua præter naturam congeratur; ſane poterit, ſi necdum illud con- " creverit, ejus concretionem ſuo interjectu prohibere : aut ſi jam concreverit; inter " ejus particulas ſe inſinuando, has ſenſim magis magisque disjungere, donec ad mi- " nimas ventum ſit, facile cum aqua permiſcendas, neque amplius internoſcendas."— 6. " In altero Hydrocephalo non ſolum disjunctionem propemodum perfectam ſed " disjunctarum particularum cum aqua permiſtionem ipſa indicabit aqua loturæ car- " nium ſimilis, præterquam et craſſum meningem nihil diſtincti in diffluente cerebro " videre licuit."

Haller, in Elem. Phyſ. L. x. § xxxix. " Quod autem, diſſoluto in aquam Cere- " bro et demum amiſſo vivatur," &c. . . . . . .

" Eo modo credibile eſt, ſenſim quidem Cerebrum contabuiſſe in aquam."

As a confequence of fuch an opinion, it fhould follow, that the Watery Liquor poffeffed the farther quality of rendering the white and opaque Medullary Subftance of the Brain tranfparent; and, on evaporating the water, the Medullary Subftance fhould remain in the form of an extract.

But, inftead of that, we do not perceive how the water effufed into the Ventricles is brought in contact with the medullary or other fubftance of the Brain, as the Ventricles are lined with thin but denfe membrane.—We do not find that we can diffolve the Medullary Subftance of the Brain in the Watery Liquor we extract from the Ventricles of the Brain of a perfon labouring under Hydrocephalus.

When we heat and evaporate the Watery Liquor collected in Hydrocephalus, we are fo far from recovering the medullary fubftance of the Brain, that very little coagulable or folid matter is found in the refiduum; for the quantity even of the coagulable lymph is lefs in this than in moft other fpecies of Dropfy *.

 Similar

* BONETI, Sep. L. i. S. 16. Ad. Obf. 12. De Hydrocephalo, "Aquæ, in "cochleari ferreo, nonnihil prunis impofuimus. Non in gelatinam concrévit, uti "aqua in ventre Hydropicorum folet, fed, poft evaporationem, fal acre reliquit."

Similar Watery Liquor, effufed in the other fpecies of Dropfy, is not found, nor fuppofed, to poffefs any fuch folvent power.

I apprehend, therefore, that this hypothefis is to be entirely rejected; and, that inftead of fuppofing that the parts of the Brain difappear becaufe they are melted down by the Water, and rendered pellucid, we are to imagine, that the parts of the Brain are carried off by the Abforbent Veffels; which are excited to unufual action, by the tenfion and irritation which the Water occafions.

In a cafe, very different from Dropfy, to which I was called, in 1784, along with Dr CHARLES WEBSTER, I have likewife feen undoubted proof, that a great part of the folid fubftance of the Brain muft have been carried away by the Abforbent Veffels. The Patient, a ftout man, about thirty years of age, had, for ten months, complained of the moft excruciating pain in the right fide of his Forehead. At laft he was feized with delirium, which terminated in ftupor and apoplexy; and in this ftate I found him. He died next day. On opening his Head, the Left Hemifphere of the Brain was found to have its ufual appearance; but the Anterior

Anterior Lobe of the Right Hemiſphere was of a deep purple colour, very conſiderably indurated, and adhered firmly to the Supra Orbitar Plate. On cutting it perpendicularly into two parts, which I preſerve, the diſtinction of Cineritious and Medullary Matter was ſcarcely obſervable; for the whole of it was of a dark purple colour, nearly uniform in texture, and had large and numerous veſſels, filled with red blood, in its compoſition reſembling the Lungs in an inflamed ſtate more than the Brain.

There was no effuſion of water or of blood, nor collection of purulent matter. It was therefore evident, that, in proportion to the enlargement of the Blood-veſſels, and perhaps increaſe of their number, there muſt have been an Abſtraction of the Cineritious and Medullary Matter made by the Abſorbent Veſſels.

As the Cortical and Medullary Subſtances of the Brain are not evidently compreſſible, it follows, that in the caſes of Sudden Apoplexy, Epilepſy, Suffocation from Noxious Vapours, Drowning, Hanging, there can be no ſuch ſenſible general Enlargement of the Blood-veſſels as has been ſuppoſed and deſcribed by Authors. But if, by long-continued intemperance,

intemperance, or other caufes, the Blood has been circulated within the Head with more than ufual violence, there may have been an increafed Abforption or Wafting of the folid Subftance of the Encephalon; and, in proportion to that, an Enlargement of the Blood-veffels, and evident Increafe of the Quantity of Blood within the Head.

CHAP.

CHAP. V.

Circumſtances enumerated, which prove, That the Solid Parts compoſing the other Organs of our Body are Abſorbed.

THAT the Solid Matter of the Brain can be carried off by the Abſorbent Veſſels, appears, at firſt ſight, an opinion ſo incredible, that I ſhall endeavour to ſupport it by the following Obſervations,—which, I apprehend, prove beyond a doubt, that the Solid as well as the Fluid Parts of Animals are under a conſtant ſtate of Change.

a. The

a. The Several Glands and Glandular Vifcera are often enlarged and indurated, remain in that ftate for a confiderable time, and fometimes return to their natural fize and recover their found ftructure.

b. Hemorrhoidal Tumours, which I have found to contain a great deal of folid matter, inftead of being entirely produced, as MORGAGNI and HALLER have affirmed *, by a varicous ftate of the Veins, after increafing to confiderable bulk, difappear almoft entirely, leaving nothing but the fkin which covered them.

c. Venereal Excrefcences, called Fici, Mori, &c. are often removed by the internal ufe of Mercury.

d. The glandular body called Thymus, generally difappears, or is abforbed, before the fixteenth year of life.

e. Where

* MORGAGNI, Ep. xxxii. 10, 11.

HALLER, El. Phyf. T. vii. lxxiv. S. iv. § xii. p. 193.

e. Where the Skin is extended, and at the ſame time irritated, by an abſceſs forming under it in the condenſed cellular ſubſtance, it is waſted, and ſometimes breaks into holes, ſeveral days before the purulent matter contained in the abſceſs is diſcharged, that is, before the matter is in contact with the ſkin.

f. In like manner, the Fleſhy Parts of the Muſcles ſometimes ſhrink greatly, loſe their red colour and fibrous appearance, and ſeem to be converted into white-coloured tough membranes. I have long had in my poſſeſſion a preparation, in which a large portion of the Apex of the Left Ventricle of the Heart of a Man has entirely loſt its Fleſhy Structure, and has the appearance of a white, tough, thin membrane. Within this part is contained a whitiſh firm Grume formed by the blood, ſuch as is found in Aneuriſmal Sacs.——In other inſtances, the whole Fleſhy Part of a Muſcle is removed, without the application to it of fluid or acrid matter, which could be ſuppoſed to have corroded or melted it down into a liquid ſtate. A remarkable example of this kind occurred about twenty years ago, in the caſe of an eminent Phyſician, Dr Au——n, whom I attended along with Dr Hay and the late Dr Hope, and who, for upwards of a year before his death, had been diſtreſſed with pains in the inteſtines. On opening his body, we found, to our ſurpriſe, that the diſtended Sigmoid Flexure of the Colon was firmly united with the Skin, and that the Abdominal Muſcles were entirely removed from a ſpace larger than the whole hand could cover.

In Old Perſons, I have repeatedly found, that the Cavities of ſome of the Burſæ Mucoſæ which are contiguous to Ligaments, communicated with the Cavities of the Joints, in conſequence of a Waſting of the Membranes of the Burſæ and Ligaments. Theſe Perſons had not, in life, complained of pain; no acrid, purulent, or other liquor, was collected; the ſides of the holes by which the communications were made, were not ragged, but ſmooth; no lacerated membranes were found floating in the Burſæ or in the Joints: The Waſte, therefore, could only have been produced by the gradual Abſorption of the Particles which had compoſed the Membranes.

g. But the moſt ſtriking proofs that the Solids may be Abſorbed, are to be drawn from attention to the Structure and Growth of the Bones, and to their Waſte by age and diſeaſe.

h. When Powder of Madder is mixed with the ordinary food of an Animal, it communicates its colour to the clear

part

part of the Blood, and ſoon thereafter the Bones are tinged. The Red Colour of the Bone, in ſome degree, depends on the Particles of the Madder mixed with the Blood in the Veſſels of the Bone; but as I have found, that the Colour is little, indeed not ſenſibly, changed by injecting pure water into the Veſſels, and waſhing the Blood out of them, it is certain, that the Colour is chiefly owing to a Red Earthy Matter which has been added to the Bones whilſt the Animal was fed with the mixture of Madder. If the Madder be withdrawn from the food of the Animal, the Red Colour diſappears, which can only be by its Abſorption.

i. The Skeleton of a very Old Perſon is ſo much Lighter than that of a middle-aged perſon of the ſame ſtature, that the difference cannot be accounted for on the common ſuppoſition that the Solids are compacted, and the Fluids alone abſorbed.

k. On comparing a conſiderable number of Sculls of very Old Perſons, with an equal number of thoſe of Middle Age, I have found, that they had loſt about Two Parts of Five of their Weight.

l. In the Jaw-bones of Old Perſons, beſides their general loſs of weight in common with the other bones, the Sockets of the Teeth, after theſe drop out, are removed entirely; ſo that the Lower Jaw-bone loſes nearly one half of its depth, and, upon the whole, more than one half of its weight.

m. In the Aneuriſm of the Arch of the Aorta, of which many caſes are in my poſſeſſion, the Sternum, the Ribs, their Cartilages, the Cartilages of the Trachea are altered in their ſhape, and waſted in their ſubſtance, long before the Blood gets into contact with them; which muſt be owing to an increaſed Abſorption.

n. In Venereal Caſes, the Bones ſometimes ſwell conſiderably, or Nodes form upon them, both of which effects are often diſperſed by Mercury.

o. In a very large collection of Morbid Bones in my poſſeſſion, whilſt, in many inſtances, their thickneſs and weight are much greater than in ſound bones, in others, their weight is greatly diminiſhed.

p. In ſome caſes of Ulcerous Caries affecting the lower end of the Tibia and Joint of the Ankle, I have found, after

ter amputation was performed, that the Bones of the Tarſus and Metatarſus, at a diſtance from the ulcer, were much Softer and Lighter than in a ſound perſon of the ſame age.

q. In Rickets, although the Bones, and particularly their Extremities, are enlarged, yet the Skeleton of a Rickety Child is commonly Lighter than that of Children of the ſame age who are killed by other diſeaſes.——In ſome caſes of Rickets, the Bones become not only thicker but heavier than in the ſound ſtate: In proof of which, I have in my poſſeſſion the Parietal Bones of a Rickety Perſon which are upwards of an inch in thickneſs.

r. In the diſeaſe called Incarnation of Bones, becauſe they are ſoft and may be cut like fleſh, the Bones become ſemitranſparent, and extremely light; and, in ſome caſes, whilſt theſe changes were going on in them, it was obſerved that the Urine depoſited a large quantity of a White Plaſtery-looking Sediment; to which is added, in one caſe of a Woman, of the name Sue, that before the diſeaſe began, ſhe had been in the habit of devouring daily a great quantity of Sea-ſalt. There can be no doubt, therefore, that, in this diſeaſe, the Earthy Matter of the Bones is carried

ried off by the Abſorbing Veſſels: In conſequence of which, thoſe Bones, or Parts of Bones, which naturally are the hardeſt, or have the greateſt quantity of Earth in their compoſition, are by this diſeaſe rendered the ſofteſt.

f. From the whole, it appears, not only, that the Solid Parts of the Body may be Abſorbed in conſequence of Diſeaſe; but, that in Health, and during the whole Courſe of Life, there is ſuch a conſtant Interchange of the Particles which compoſe the Solids, by means of the Veſſels which Secrete and Abſorb, as to render it doubtful whether a ſingle Atom remains in our Bodies which formed a part of them ſome years ago.

CHAP.

CHAP. VI.

At what Time the Circumſtances enumerated in the laſt Chapter were firſt taught by the Author.

OF late years, the Abſorption of the Solid Parts of Animals has been mentioned by a few Writers who have publiſhed in London: And as Mr JOHN HUNTER has been quoted by ſome of them, as the Author of this Doctrine, I muſt here obſerve, that ſo far back as the year 1759, and ever ſince that time, I have mentioned, in different parts of my annual Courſe of Lectures in this Univerſity, all the Circumſtances above mentioned which relate to the Bones, and likewiſe

likewiſe ſeveral of the Circumſtances which appeared to prove an Abſorption of the other Solid Parts; and, particularly, I endeavoured to explain, on this principle, the Changes which are produced on the Sternum and Ribs by Aneuriſm, which Dr WILLIAM HUNTER, at that time, accounted for, on the erroneous ſuppoſition, that theſe Bones were melted down by the current and ſolvent power of the Blood. See Med. Obſ. and Inq. vol. i. 1757, p. 344. "But "in this caſe," ſays he, "the appearance was rather as if "the Blood had inſenſibly diſſolved and waſhed away the "Subſtance of the Bone, making greateſt havock in the "ſofteſt part of the Bone, as we ſee in ſtones of unequal "texture that have been long waſhed by a dropping, or a "ſtream of water. Has the Bone that property which ſome "have aſcribed to it, of diſſolving Bony Matter?" &c.

It is plain, then, either, that Mr JOHN HUNTER had not, at that time, propoſed the Doctrine of the Abſorption of Oſſeous Matter; or, if he did ſo, that his Brother was ignorant of it, or paid no regard to it.

When, near twenty years thereafter, Mr JOHN HUNTER mentioned ſuch an opinion in his Lectures, it appears, from the teſtimony of a very ſenſible and ingenious gentleman, (Dr

(Dr WINTERBOTTOM), who attended him then, and who, in his Thefis, has fhewn his difpofition to do him juftice, that he refted his opinion chiefly, if not folely, on the circumftance, that in Growing Animals the Medullary Canal is enlarged in its diameter; which he took for granted muft be owing to an Abforption of the Internal Layers of the Bone, whilft new Layers were adding to its external part; not knowing that the celebrated DU HAMEL has, upwards of half a century ago, proved by the following fimple and decifive experiment, That the Diameter of a Bone, as well as that of its Medullary Canal, is increafing in Growing Animals, by an Extenfion of the feveral Layers which compofe it. See Mem. de l'Acad. des Sc. 1743, p. 102. "J'entourai l'Os d'un Pigeonneau Vivant avec un Anneau de "fil d'argent, qui étoit placé fous les Tendons et fur le Periofte. Je laiffai là cet Anneau, pour reconnoître ce qui "arriveroit aux couches Offeufes déjà formées, fuppofé "qu'elles vinffent à s'etendre; car je penfois que mon Anneau étoit plus fort qu'il ne falloit pour refifter à l'effort "que ces lames Offeufes feroient pour s'etendre. Il refiftoit "en effet; et les couches Offeufes, qui n'étoient pas encore "fort dures, ne pouvant s'etendre vis-à-vis l'Anneau, fe coupperent. Ce qui prouve bien l'Extenfion des Couches Offeufes, c'eft qu'ayant diffequé la partie, je trouvai, que le

" Diametre de l'Anneau n'étoit pas plus grand que celui du " Canal Medullaire."——To ſhew ſtill more clearly, that Mr JOHN HUNTER had built his opinion on an erroneous foundation, I have remarked, in many Diſeaſed Bones in my poſſeſſion, in which the Thickneſs of the Bones is greatly increaſed, that the Medullary Canal is much diminiſhed. ——From this, and from DU HAMEL's experiment, then, we may obſerve, that the Plates of the Bones may be extended in all directions, or, that they grow in length, breadth, and thickneſs.

Dr WINTERBOTTOM, after attending Mr JOHN HUNTER's Lectures, ſtudied the uſual number of years in this Univerſity, and received the Degree of Doctor of Medicine, in 1781, after publiſhing an excellent Diſſertation, De Vaſis Abſorbentibus.

In this, p. 27. he writes as follows:

" § 34. Abſorbentia, Fluida ſorbere, jamdiu notum; gloria autem monſtrandi ea Solida quoque haurire, penes " MONRO Anatomicum peritiſſimum eſt. In hanc ſententiam, uti jamdudum in Prælectionibus prædicavit, multis " argumentis adductus ibat: Sed præſertim, quia Thymum " glandulam

" glandulam evanefcere ; Offa Senis multo leviora quam Ju-
" venis effe ; Terram Rubram, quam Rubia Tinctorum in
" Offa infert, poft aliquod tempus auferri ; etiamque variis
" in morbis Offa mollia, diftorta, fere pellucida, et levia, de-
" venire ; imo, aliquot in exemplis, infolitam quantitatem
" Sedimenti Albidi, Terræ Offium fimillime, in Urina fuiffe
" inventam, — animadvertit.

" In Prælectionibus, de eadem re, obfervavit cl. JOANNES
" HUNTER, " Quamvis difficile comprehenfu fit quomodo
" Vafa poffint Solida amovere, æque tamen difficile compre-
" henfu quomodo ea formare poffint, quod nihilo feciùs ferè
" omnes credunt."

" § 35. Solida non minus quam Fluida abforberi, pro
" certo affirmare haud cunctor ; namque Offa Hominis, me-
" dia ætate, plus Ponderis quam Senilia, æque ampla ha-
" bent. Quibufdam in exemplis quoque Atrophiæ et Tabis,
" partem offium effe abforptam, inter Auctores omnes con-
" venit.

" § 36. Hanc rem JOANNES HUNTER quàm pulcherrimè
" fic illuftrat, (*in Prælectionibus) : " In Offe Femoris In-

H 2 " fantis,

" ſantis, Cavitas initio perexigua eſt; corpore autem creſ-
" cente, amplior evadit: Ita, dum Arteriæ Terram Oſſis
" externæ parti adjiciunt, Abſorbentia eam internè ad-
" imunt."

Dr WINTERBOTTOM adds, in a Note †, " Hoc aliter ex-
" plicari poſſe equidem non nego; ſed opinio modò poſi-
" ta, etſi non omninò certa, pulchra ſaltem mihi vide-
" tur."

CHAP.

CHAP. VII.

Of the Cure of Internal Hydrocephalus by Medicines.

AS, probably, the Particles composing the Solids of our Body are dissolved by Secreted Fluids, or reduced to a Fluid State before they be fit for being absorbed; and as, therefore, the Waste of the Solids, by the Absorption of them, must be performed by a much more complex process than that of Fluids; we should, after finding proof that the Cineritious and Medullary Matter of the Brain can be removed by it, be apt, at first sight, to suppose, that the Internal Hydrocephalus could be easily cured by Medicine. But, when

when we reflect, that the Diſtenſion and Irritation, which create the unuſual exertion of the Abſorbent Syſtem, ſeem to operate ſtill more powerfully on the Secerning Veſſels, and that whilſt the Abſorbents are preying on the Solid Matter of the Brain, the Effuſion of the Watery Liquor is increaſing rapidly, we begin to perceive, that the Cure muſt be much more difficult than we had ſuppoſed it to be: And, as we find, by experience, that Irritation greatly increaſes the diſcharge from exhaling veſſels, I have often thought, that the ſingular Senſibility of the Parts of the Brain, highly excited by the Diſtenſion of its Ventricles in Hydrocephalus, muſt, in it, render the chance of Cure far leſs than it is in other ſpecies of Encyſted Dropſy.

Of late years, Mercury has been much extolled for the cure of Hydrocephalus Internus; and various caſes of ſucceſs with it, even after the diſeaſe had made conſiderable progreſs, have been publiſhed.

I ſhall ſubjoin a Summary Account of the Caſes in which I have made trial of it.

Since the month of Auguſt 1779, I have attended Twenty-two Patients, labouring under Internal Hydrocephalus, to whom

I

I have given Mercury. —— Of theſe, Fifteen were Males, and Seven Females. —— Twelve of them were under Seven years of age: Nine of them were from Eight to Fourteen years of age: One was Twenty-three years old. —— Four of them lived Five Days only after I was called: Nine of them ſurvived Seven or Eight Days: Three of them ſurvived Ten Days: Five of them ſurvived Thirteen or Fourteen Days: One, Six years of age, ſurvived Four Months, without any ſenſible Enlargement of his Head.

In treating theſe caſes, I generally began with the application of Leeches to the Temples. I then gave Calomel, in ſuch quantity as to act as a briſk purgative. I applied a large Bliſter to the Top of the Head. In ſome caſes, I kept a portion of the bliſtered part open as an Iſſue. In others, I applied Bliſters in ſucceſſion to different parts of the Head. In all of them, I directed, that ſtrong Mercurial Ointment ſhould be carefully rubbed upon the Skin of the Legs or Arms, morning and evening: And, in ſeverals, I added Doſes of Calomel by the Mouth; taking care not to give ſo much of it as to occaſion purging.——In ſome caſes, I combined the Powder of Squills with the Calomel; and in a few, the Powder of the Digitalis Purpurea.

In Four of theſe caſes, the Gums became Red, but with little ſwelling: In Four others, the Gums were not only Red, but conſiderably ſwelled. In Two caſes, there was a free Salivation. In the Boy, ſix years old, who ſurvived four months, a profuſe Salivation was kept up for ſeven weeks; yet, after his death, Eight Ounces of Water were found in the Ventricles of the Brain, by Mr GULLON, Surgeon in Dunfermline, under whoſe care he was after the Salivation.—— In none of the other caſes, were the effects of the Mercury diſtinguiſhable.

As, in the greater number of the above caſes, the diſeaſe had made conſiderable progreſs before I was called; and as moſt of the Patients ſurvived but for a ſhort time thereafter; the Effects which the Mercury may have, if given on the firſt appearance of the ſymptoms, are by no means fully determined. And, as I have repeatedly found, in other dangerous ſpecies of the Natural Encyſted Dropſy, particularly in Hydrothorax and Aſcites, that Mercury, combined with Squills or other diuretic medicines, in ſuch quantity as to ſalivate in a ſlight degree, contributed much to the relief or cure of the Patient; I would recommend the farther trial of it in Hydrocephalus. At the ſame time, conſidering

conſidering the importance, ſenſibility, and delicate texture, of the parts which are affected, and total failure in the caſes I have deſcribed; I cannot help ſuſpecting, that ſeveral late Writers are much too ſanguine in their expectation of removing Hydrocephalus by the uſe of Mercury.

CHAP. VIII.

Of the Cure of Hydrocephalus Internus by Chirurgical Operation.

FOUR different States of the Diſeaſe may occur, which we ſhall conſider ſeparately.

1. If, when the diſeaſe began, it was not attended with acute pain, and the other common ſymptoms; for I think there can be no doubt that the Patient muſt ſuffer much more diſtreſs when the Water is collected within and diſtends the Ven-

 tricles,

tricles, than where it is effuſed on the External Surface of the Brain: and if, from a very evident fluctuation of the Water, chiefly at the Bregma, it is ſuppoſed, that the Water is ſituated immediately within the Dura Mater, between it and the Surfaces of the Brain, Cerebellum and Spinal Marrow: we ought to puncture the Dura Mater; as this can be done without danger, may give immediate relief, and may have ſome chance of producing a cure. The Dura Mater ought to be punctured cautiouſly with a Lancet, at the ſide of the Bregma, or as far as poſſible from the Superior Longitudinal Sinus.

In my Book on the Nervous Syſtem, Chap. iv. Sect. 3. I have given the hiſtory of one attempt of this kind, which I directed; and ſhall here refer the Reader to it.

2. If the Water be collected, in ſmall quantity, within the Ventricles, which is almoſt always the caſe in the Acute Hydrocephalus, the deep Wound of the Subſtance of the Brain, which muſt be inflicted in order to reach the cavity of the Ventricles, would probably prove fatal directly, or indirectly by exciting inflammation: or, if it ſhould

neither

neither immediately prove fatal, nor excite inflammation, the Water would ſoon be again collected; and, of courſe, the diſeaſe would, ere long, terminate in death.

3. In the Chronic Species of Internal Hydrocephalus, where the Head is enlarged by Water, which has been gradually collecting, and is ſtill entirely confined within the Ventricles of the Brain, ſome Authors have propoſed, and, in a few caſes, have ventured, to diſcharge the Water by puncture with a Trocar. But, within a few hours after the operation, every one of their Patients died *.

Upon

* Ep. Ferdinandes, Hiſt. 1611 "Hydrocephalum infantis incidit, funeſto "eventu."

G. Fabricius, Cent. iii. Obſ. 17. "Ab Hydrocephalo inciſo, aperto Bregmate, "mors."

D. Panarolus, in Iatrolog. "In Hydrocephalo, a perforatione cranii mors."

Wepfer,

Upon the whole: When we conſider the various dangers which muſt ariſe from the puncture of the ſubſtance of the Brain; from the unequal bending, preſſure, and perhaps laceration of parts, which muſt happen when the Brain collapſes; from the admiſſion of the air; from the impoſſibility of adapting the Cranium exactly to the Brain for its ſupport, by the application of any bandage; — no prudent Surgeon will embark himſelf in ſuch an attempt, — "Ne, "quem ſervare non potuit, occidiſſe videatur."

---

4. If the Water, after having been collected and confined within the Ventricles of the Brain, ſhall have made its way out of theſe, in conſequence of the deſtruction of ſome of the Solid Subſtance of the Brain by the Abſorbent Veſſels, ſo as to be lodged, in part, between the Outer Surface of the

---

Wepfer, Obſ. 49. "Hydrocephalus, in Puella quinque annorum, infeliciter "ſectus."

"Muraltus fruſtrà tentavit curationem Hydrocephali inciſi."

Le Cat. Phil. Tr. Vol. xlvii. Art. 40.

the Brain and the Dura Mater, although it may be dischar-ged by a puncture of the Common Teguments and Dura Mater only; yet, as the substance of the Brain has been materially injured by the disease, the case is evidently, in all other respects, more desperate than the former.

THE END OF TREATISE FIRST.

MISCELLANEOUS

OBSERVATIONS

ON THE

STRUCTURE AND FUNCTIONS

OF THE

EYES.

BY

ALEXANDER MONRO, M. D.

PROFESSOR OF MEDICINE, ANATOMY, AND SURGERY,

IN THE UNIVERSITY OF EDINBURGH.

EDINBURGH:

PRINTED BY ADAM NEILL AND COMPANY.

1797.

A Table of the Contents of Treatise II.

CHAP.

TREATISE SECOND:

OF THE EYES.

INTRODUCTION.

IN this Paper, I ſhall briefly ſtate ſome material circumſtances, reſpecting the Structure and Functions of the Eyes, which have eſcaped the obſervation of Authors; or, concerning which, erroneous opinions have, I apprehend, been entertained by them: And I ſhall begin with Remarks on the Humours of the Eye, and from theſe ſhall proceed outwards, as I have found that a Demonſtration or Deſcription in this order is the moſt intelligible.

CHAP. I.

Of the Capſule of the Vitreous Humour.

THE Capſule of the Vitreous Humour, from the Bottom of the Eyeball till it gets forwards as far as to the Roots of the Ciliary Proceſſes, is ſo extremely thin and delicate, that it can ſcarcely be demonſtrated by Diſſection; and, ſo far, it has very little adheſion to the Retina which covers it.

Within the Roots of the Ciliary Proceſſes, it adheres cloſely to the Retina; and, a little farther forwards, it ſeems to divide into two diſtinct Layers. The External continues to be glued to the Retina, and accompanies it to its termina-

K 2 tion,

tion, which we ſhall find to be in the Forepart of the Capſule of the Cryſtalline Lens, about one-twentieth of an inch from its outer edge: The Internal Layer adheres firmly to the Vitreous Humour, till this is connected with the poſterior part of the Capſule of the Lens, at the like diſtance, nearly, of one-twentieth of an inch from its outer edge; and at the diſtance, therefore, of one-tenth of an inch from the connexion of its Anterior Layer and Retina with the Lens. The outer edge, therefore, of the Cryſtalline Lens, covered with its proper Capſule only, occupies a ſpace nearly one-tenth of an inch in breadth, between the two Layers of the Capſule of the Vitreous Humour.

The Anterior Layer of the Vitreous Humour being fixed to the Cryſtalline Lens, at the diſtance, nearly, of one-tenth of an inch from the attachment of its Poſterior Layer,— a Canal, bounded by the Two Layers of the Vitreous Humour, and by the edge of the Cryſtalline Lens, as its baſis, is formed, which was diſcovered by Dr Petit, and is named after him *. Air, blown into this ſpace, paſſes, of courſe, around

* Mem. de l'Acad. des Sciences, 1726.

around the Cryſtalline Lens. Each of the Two Layers of the Capſule of the Vitreous Humour, is tougher than the poſterior part of the Capſule, and adheres firmly to the Capſule of the Lens *.

CHAP.

* See Table I. Fig. 3. 4. 5.

CHAP. II.

Of the Cryſtalline Lens.

SECT. I.

Of the Capſule of the Cryſtalline Lens.

THE Capſule of the Cryſtalline Lens, is of conſiderable thickneſs; but has little toughneſs, or is eaſily cut or lacerated.

The Capſule of the Vitreous Humour, by its diviſion into the Two Layers I have deſcribed, has been ſuppoſed to form it *. But this is an erroneous opinion; for, it is not only much

* WINSLOW, Traité de la Tête, 235. " La Capſule Cryſtallaine eſt formée " par la Duplicature de la Tunique Vitrée, comme j'ai dit, 229."

much Thicker than the Capſule of the Vitreous Humour, but is found on the Outer Edge of the Lens, covering that part of it which lies between the Anterior and Poſterior Layers of the Vitreous Capſule, and which is not covered by theſe.

Oculiſts, founding on the Diviſion of the Capſule of the Vitreous Humour into Two Layers, which paſs to the fore and back parts of the Capſule of the Lens, have conſidered theſe as Membranes ſuperadded, and looſely connected to the Capſule of the Lens; and therefore pretend to detach the Lens, in its proper Capſule, from the Poſterior Layer of the Capſule of the Vitreous Humour, without lacerating it, or breaking the Subſtance of the Vitreous Humour *. But, in fact, Both Layers of the Capſule of the Vitreous Humour are ſo intimately connected to, and incorporated with, the Capſule of the Lens, that the Poſterior Part of the Capſule of the Lens cannot be ſeparated from that of the Vitreous Humour, without tearing it, and, with it, the Subſtance of the Vitreous Humour.

SECT.

* Mr. du Wenzel, on the Cataract, Sect. xxvi.

SECT. II.

Of the Structure of the Body of the Cryſtalline Lens, and Whether the Fibres which enter into its compoſition are Muſcular?

IT has been long known, that the Cryſtalline Lens conſiſts of Lamellæ, which are very ſoft and tender on its ſurface, but become firmer, tougher, and heavier, as we approach to its centre; and that the Lamellæ are compoſed of Fibres.

LEEUWENHOEK, who firſt obſerved the Fibrous Structure of the Lens, has deſcribed them as diſpoſed in a very complex and regular manner, and he ſuppoſed them to be Muſcular; and this deſcription and opinion have of late been revived.

I had, many years ago, examined and demonſtrated the Fibrous Structure of the Lens, in the different Claſſes of Animals, which I mentioned in my Book on Fiſhes, Ch. XI.; and, lately, I have repeated my obſervations, with the aid of the Microſcope, without finding that the Fibres are diſpoſed in the regular manner which has been deſcribed and delineated with ſo much ſeeming accuracy, or that they can be at all ſeen till after the Lens is torn or cut: and, beſides their Want of Reſemblance to Muſcle and Tendon, the following arguments appear to me to render the opinion of their being Muſcular extremely queſtionable.

1. After the Cryſtalline Lens is extracted, the Eye, aſſiſted by a Common Lens, ſeems capable of adapting itſelf to different diſtances. In Two Caſes I examined, above twenty years ago, it appeared to be ſo: At the ſame time, I muſt acknowledge I could not truſt ſo entirely to the report of the patients as to be fully convinced of this.

2. I ſhall, in a following part of this Paper, endeavour to prove, that we poſſeſs other means of accommodating the Eye to objects placed at different diſtances.

3. The External Lamellæ of the Lens, and the Matter which connects the Lens with its Capſule, are ſo extremely Soft, that ſuch a degree of muſcular action of theſe Fibres as could occaſion any alteration of its general ſhape, could ſcarcely fail to lacerate the external part of the Lens, and to detach it from its Capſule.

4. In

4. In Fishes, where these Fibres are more manifest than in other Animals, as the Crystalline Lens is nearly spherical, and the Matter composing it nearly incompressible, the Fibres composing its Lamellæ, although they possessed a Muscular Power, could neither change its Spherical Figure, nor render it more Convex by lessening the Diameter or Bulk of the Sphere.

SECT. III.

Of the Refractive Power of the Crystalline Lens.

It has been very generally supposed, by Anatomists and by Opticians, that the Refractive Power of the Crystalline Lens, compared with that of Water, is proportioned nearly to its density; or, that its power exceeds that of Water somewhat, on account of the Inflammable Matter which enters into its composition *. But different considerations, and particular-

 ly,

* Haller, in Elem. Phys. Vol. v. Lib. xvi. p. 402. "Parvam esse qua aquam "superat, prærogativam, nuperi fatentur. Erit tamen aliqua, et ex ponderis ra- "tione,

ly, that the rays of light cannot be refracted on entering the Cornea in Fiſhes, and therefore that their Cryſtalline Lens, which is not more diſtant from the Retina than in Land Animals, muſt poſſeſs much greater power of Refraction, — having led me to ſuſpect an error in the common opinion, and to put this highly curious point of Phyſiology to the teſt of experiment, I diſcovered, That the Spherical Nucleus of the Cryſtalline Lens of the Cod, which, in ſpecific gravity, is to Water nearly as 6 to 5, and to common white Glaſs as 3 only to 10, collects the Light ſo much more powerfully than Water or Glaſs does, that its Focus is not more than one-ſixth part of its Diameter diſtant from its Surface; whereas the Focus of the Rays collected by a Glaſs Sphere, is at the diſtance of one-fourth of the Diameter of the Sphere; and the Focus of the Rays collected by

" tione, quæ tamen fere ſit ut 11 ad 10, et particularum inflammabilium. An-
" gulum incidentiæ radii ex humore aqueo in lentem venientis, ad angulum re-
" fractionis, facit uti 87 ad 85, cl. PORTERFIELD: Eandem rationem æſtimat
" cl. PEMBERTONUS, uti 13 ad 12; et uti 21 ad 20, cl. WINTRINGHAM." And Dr PORTERFIELD adds, " This is a ſurpriſingly ſmall refraction, and yet it is as " certain as any thing in EUCLID, that it can be no greater."

by a Sphere of Water, is diſtant from it one-half of its Diameter *.

On performing a ſimilar experiment with the Human Cryſtalline Lens, I found, that the Focus, of parallel rays of light falling on it, is at the diſtance of three-eighths of an inch from its Centre.

But, although this ſhews, that its powers are far inferior to thoſe of the Lens of the Fiſh, and even to thoſe of Glaſs, which, of the ſame ſize and ſhape, would collect the light at the diſtance of a quarter of an inch †; yet, as the Specific Weight of the Human Lens does not exceed that of Water above a tenth part, its powers are much greater than have been ſuppoſed by Authors; and the Focus formed by the Human Lens, will be found to be ſituated, nearly, half-way between thoſe produced by Glaſs and Water.

CHAP.

* For a more particular Account of my Experiments, I ſhall refer to my Book on the Structure and Phyſiology of Fiſhes, 1785,—Chap. xi.

† In this calculation, I ſuppoſe that the Radius of the Sphere of which the Anterior Part of the Lens is a portion, is 7¼ lines in length, and that of its Poſterior Part 5 lines only.

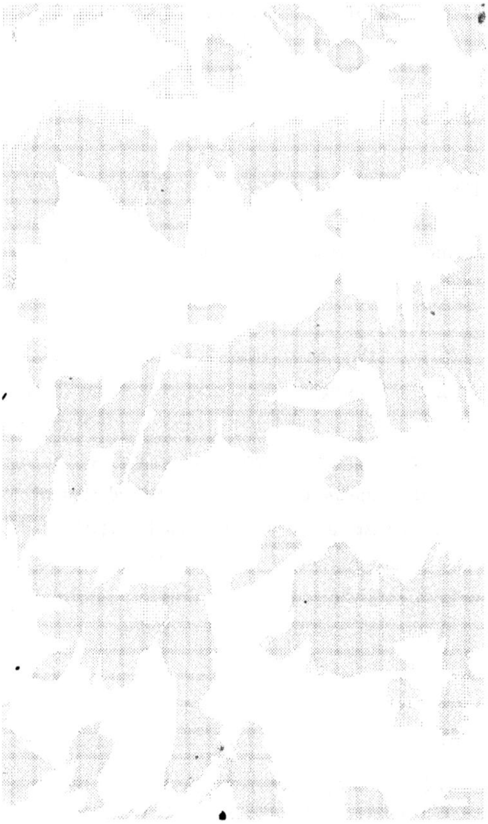

CHAP. III.

Of the Optic Nerves and Retina.

THE Optic Nerves have, in their whole courſe, leſs appearance of a Fibrous Structure than perhaps any other pair of Nerves in the Human Body.

SECT. I.

HENCE, although it appears to me evident, that the Medullary Matter of the Right Nerve is incorporated with that of the Left, where they are connected within the Head, yet I have found it very difficult, if not impoſſible, to determine in in what proportion of parts the mixture is made, or to trace either of the Nerves, with certainty, from its Origin to its Termination in the Retina.

SECT. II.

MARIOTTE, above a century ago, has, by an ingenious experiment, proved, that we are infenfible of an object if its picture falls on the Entrance of the Optic Nerve into the Eyeball. On repeating this experiment, many years ago, I found, that the Diameter of the Object which difappears is very nearly equal to one-ninth part of our diftance from it; or, that, at the diftance of Nine Feet from a wall, a Circle One Foot in Diameter is loft. If, therefore, we fuppofe the Human Eye to be One Inch or Twelve Lines in Diameter, and that the Rays of Light, iffuing from the Object, decuffate about the Centre of the Cryftalline Lens, which is nearly Three Lines behind the Cornea, or Nine Lines from the Retina, — the infenfible Spot on the Bottom of the Eye will be One Line in Diameter; and with this calculation I found that the actual meafurement of the Medullary Part of the Optic Nerve agrees very nearly.

I

I next found, that an object begins to disappear, when the point to which the Eye is directed, is One-fourth of the distance of the Eye from it; and hence, upon the supposition above stated, the Axis of the Eyeball will be found to be Two Lines and a Quarter from the Outer Side of the Optic Nerve, and Two Lines and Three Quarters from its Centre.

SECT. III.

When the Nerves, after entering the Eyeballs, form the Retina, their Colour is changed from White to Cineritious; but no Fibres are to be seen in the Human Retina, even with the Microscope; but the whole appears to be composed of an Uniform Pulpy Matter, on the Outer Side of which, chiefly, Vessels are dispersed, supported, as I suppose, by a Membrane the same with or analogous to the Pia Mater. The term *Retina* is therefore improper, where it is applied to express a Network or Fibrous Texture.

SECT. IV.

Of the Termination of the Retina.

NOT long after I began to ſtudy Anatomy, finding very contradictoy accounts of the Termination of the Retina, given by the moſt eminent Authors *, and even by the ſame Authors,

---

* WINSLOW, Traité de la Tête, 237.: "C'eſt peut-être cette continuation "qui fait quelquefois paroître les Feuillets ou Proceſſes Ciliaires comme revetus "d'une Pellicule Blanchâtre; et c'eſt peut-être, auſſi, ce qui augmente l'epaiſſeur "de la portion anterieure de la Capſule Cryſtallaine." Yet, in p. 231. he deſcribes the Black Paint of the Choroid Coat as connected with the Capſule of the Vitreous Humour, inſtead of the Retina: "Les Sillons Rayonnés de la Tunique "Vitrée ſont tout à fait Noirs."

HALLER, Pr. Lin. DXV.: "Ubi vero Retina ad Proceſſus Ciliares pervenit, "ſequitur eorum ductum, et ad Lentem properat, in hujus Capſulam innata, et "huic obducta, ſi fides et aliorum cl. Virorum et meis experimentis haberi poteſt: "neque enim de eo fine in Quadrupedibus conſtat." But, in a later Work, he expreſſes his doubts of the accuracy of the above deſcription: El. Phyſ. Lib. xvi. p. 388. "Omnibus perpenſis, amplio, ei ſententiæ propior quæ Membranulam a "Retina diverſam, inter Uveam et Vitream, ad Lentem producit."

Authors, as Drs HALLER and WINSLOW, I examined this matter with ſome care in the Human Eye; and it then appeared to me, that the Retina terminated abruptly about the Root of the Ciliary Proceſſes, reſembling the Brim of a Tea-Cup: And, as the opinion of WINSLOW, FERREIN, and, at that time, of Dr HALLER, that it was fixed to and covered the Cryſtalline Lens, appeared to me incredible, becauſe it would have been ſtruck with the Light, before this was collected into a Focus or Picture; and as a Figure, publiſhed, ſome time thereafter, by the generally accurate ZINN*, ſeemed to correſpond with what I had ſeen, I proſecuted the ſubject with leſs attention than perhaps I ſhould otherwiſe have done.

Lately, I aſked the favour of my very dexterous and accurate Aſſiſtant, Mr FYFE, to repeat the diſſection of the Eye, in the Ox as well as in the Human Body, and to draw a Figure of the Termination of the Retina. His firſt Figure

* ZINN, Tab. ii. Fig. 1. and in Cap. iii. p. 116. lin. 13. "Ad Originem "Proceſſuum Ciliarium, non ſenſim evaneſcere, ſed Fine ubique æquali et accuratè limitato terminari."

correfponded with what I had obferved: But he told me, afterwards, That, on being ftill more cautious in his diffection, the Retina appeared to him to be continued on the Inner Side of the Ciliary Proceffes, and to terminate in the Outer Edge of the Cryftalline Lens. On reviewing the fubject, I obferved, beyond all doubt, that this is the cafe; and likewife difcovered the caufes of the error into which I had fallen with Dr ZINN. In the firft place, When the Continuation of the Choroid Coat and Ciliary Proceffes is lifted up, the Black Paint, which lines thefe, adheres to and conceals the Retina. In the next place, The Retina has fo much fupport from the Paint on its Outer Side, and fuch a degree of Adhefion, firft to the Capfule of the Vitreous Humour, and then to the Edge of the Lens, and has fo little Connection to the Choroid Coat behind the Root of the Ciliary Proceffes, that, in the courfe of the diffection, a flight Preffure being made, the Retina is lacerated, and appears to terminate abruptly at the Root of the Ciliary Proceffes.

To fhew the Termination of the Retina in the Outer Edge of the Cryftalline Lens, let the Eye be laid on the Cornea, and a Circular Cut then made, through all the Coats of the Eye and Vitreous Humour, behind the Ciliary Circle; the

the Retina will then be feen, lining the Black Paint upon the Ciliary Proceffes, and paffing from thefe to the Lens.

Next, let the Cornea and Sclerotic be taken off, the Iris cut away, and the Ciliary Proceffes raifed off from the Paint which lines them and fticks to the Anterior Part of the Retina; and then, with a very foft Pencil, dipt in water, let the Black Paint be brufhed off, and the whole Courfe of the Retina will be feen diftinctly.

On examining the Retina with ftill greater accuracy, it appears, that it has exactly the fame Number of Folds or Doublings that the Choroid Coat has; for it enters Double between the Ciliary Proceffes, nearly in the fame way that the Pia Mater enters into the Furrows of the Brain. The Furrows and Doublings of the Retina, which, if we are to ufe the favourite term of *Ciliary*, may be called its Ciliary Proceffes, make an impreffion on the Anterior Part of the Vitreous Humour.

I have already obferved, that the Black Paint lining the Ciliary Proceffes of the Choroid Coat, has a confiderable adhefion to the Retina, which is Thinner here than on the Pofterior Part of the Vitreous Humour; and, on its Inner

Side,,

Side, the Retina adheres ſtill more firmly to the Coat of the Vitreous Humour, which is much Tougher here than it is where it covers the Back Part of the Vitreous Humour. At laſt, the Extremities of its Ciliary Proceſſes divide into a ſtill greater Number of Parts or Fibres, reſembling the ſmall Branches of Nerves in other places of the Body, which are cloſely connected to the Fore Part of the Capſule of the Lens, about One-twentieth of an Inch diſtant from its Outer Edge, or Place where the Anterior and Poſterior Plano-convex Lenſes which form it, are joined together. After which, theſe Fibres either terminate, or become ſuddenly ſo pellucid, that it is impoſſible to trace them farther; and it is ſurely highly improbable that they form an External Coat to the Capſule of the Lens, as WINSLOW, FERREIN, and HALLER, ſuppoſed, or that their Continuation on it aſſiſts in Viſion, as the Rays of Light are not ſo fully collected upon the Capſule of the Lens as to form a diſtinct Picture, and we farther obſerve, that when a Cataract is very opake, the Light which falls on the Capſule of the Lens gives no diſtinct idea of objects.

The Retina, at its connection with the Vitreous Humour and Cryſtalline, is remarkably Tougher than it is in any other part; or it ſeems to adhere there, to the Anterior Layer of the

the Capſule of the Vitreous Humour, by Cellular Threads, or perhaps by the Pia Mater, which, as I have elſewhere endeavoured to prove, accompanies the Nerves in their whole progreſs.

In the ſeveral Figures of Table Firſt, and Table Firſt *, the Courſe and Termination of the Retina are accurately repreſented; and the Reader may now conſult the Explanation given of theſe Tables.

In conſequence of the Termination of the Retina being extended to the Cryſtalline Lens, it is evident, that, in Couching, the Surgeon muſt, before he reaches the Lens, wound the Retina with his Needle; and if he afterwards depreſſes the Capſule along with the Body of the Lens, or if a Needle is paſſed around the Lens in order to detach it from the neighbouring parts, as has been adviſed †, the Anterior Edge of the Retina muſt be lacerated, and very much injured.

As

† Mr. du Wenzel junior, on the Cataract, Sect. xvi.

As the Rays of Light cannot be directly collected, ſo as to form a diſtinct Picture on that part of the Retina which lines the Ciliary Circle and Ciliary Proceſſes, there is perhaps reaſon to ſuſpect, that the Light which is reflected from the Picture formed at the Bottom of the Eye, does not aſſiſt Viſion, by giving a Second Stroke to that part of the Retina on which the diſtinct Picture is formed,—which ſeems to be the idea of Authors; for ſuch a Second and Poſterior Stroke would have nearly or exactly the ſame effect as the Firſt: But rather, that we receive, on the Anterior Part of the Retina, lining the Ciliary Circle and Roots of the Ciliary Proceſſes, a Second and very different kind of Impulſe, by the Light reflected from the Bottom of the Eye to this part, by which we ſee and judge better of the object.

This ſuppoſition ſeems to be ſtrongly ſupported by the general obſervation, that the Paint lining the Choroid Coat at the Bottom of the Eye, which has been called *Tapetum*, is remarkably Bright, and fit for the Reflection of Light in thoſe Animals which ſeek their food in the Night-time, when ſuch an aid is evidently moſt neceſſary.

The

The Analogy of the Cochlea of the Ear, which receives One Impulſe through the Chain of Bones connected to the Membrane of the Oval Hole, and Another by the Membrane of the Foramen Rotundum, ſupports this Opinion.

CHAP. IV.

Of the Choroid Coat and Ciliary Proceſſes.

IN Man, and, ſo far as I have obſerved, in all the *Genera* of the Mammalia, Birds, Amphibia, and Fiſhes, the Choroid Coat and Ciliary Proceſſes conſiſt of a Vaſcular Coat lined with Paint: But, in one *Species*, the White Rabbit, I have found, that the Paint is wanting *, and the ſame thing is true of their Iris; and hence their Eyes appear Red; becauſe the Blood circulating in the Vaſcular Part of the Choroid, is ſeen through the Humours. It is probable, that in other *Species* or Varieties of Animals in which the Eyes appear very Red, a ſimilar Defect of the Paint will be diſcovered.

* Book on Fiſhes, Chap. xii.

I have already obſerved, that the Colour of the Paint is Brighteſt, and moſt fit to reflect Light, in thoſe Animals which ſeek their food in the Night-time: But, in all Animals which have the Paint, it is found to be Black where it lines the Ciliary Circle and Proceſſes, or where it covers the Anterior Part and Termination of the Retina; in order, I ſuppoſe, to ſuffocate the Rays of Light which are reflected from the Bottom of the Eye upon this part of the Retina: And this ſeems likewiſe to confirm what I have alleged, that no advantage in Viſion is to be derived from Light ſtriking firſt the Inner-ſide, and then being reflected upon the Outer-ſide of the ſame part of the Retina.

When the Paint is carefully waſhed off from the Inner-ſide of the Choroid Coat, we ſee evidently, that the Ciliary Proceſſes are formed by the Continuation of the Choroid Coat, folded ſeventy or eighty times, ſo as to occupy a ſmaller Circle.

The Ciliary Circle, and Roots of the Ciliary Proceſſes, are firmly glued to the Anterior Part of the Retina, almoſt as far as to its Termination, or Inſertion in the Outer Edge of the Lens: But the Points or Terminations of the Ciliary Proceſſes float looſe in the Poſterior Chamber of the Aqueous Humour,

Humour, and have no direct Connexion with the Lens. ZINN, who obferved that the Terminations of the Ciliary Proceffes were not connected with the Lens *, concluded therefore, that the Inner Parts of the Ciliary Proceffes were inferted into the Capfule of the Vitreous Humour †: But I have already obferved, that the Anterior Part of the Retina reaches to the Edge of the Lens, or intervenes between the Ciliary Proceffes and Vitreous Humour.

It appears therefore, That the Ciliary Proceffes do not form a complete Septum between the Aqueous and Vitreous Humours; and, That the Capfule of the Cryftalline Lens is not fupported in its place by the Terminations of the Ciliary Proceffes of the Choroid Coat in it; but that it owes its Support to the intimate Union of its Pofterior Part with the Pofterior Layer of the Capfule of the Vitreous Humour, and to

* See ZINN, Chap. ii. p. 66. "Ipfa tamen illa extrema libera, ad Lentem "non folum pertingant, fed etiam ultra ejus Circulum maximum progreffa, &c. "fine pendulo libero, &c. terminantur."

† ZINN, Chap. ii. p. 78. "Vitreo arctiffimè funt juncti."

to the Infertion of the Anterior Layer of the Capfule of the Vitreous Humour and Retina into it, near to its Circumference.

Whilft the Retina, by the Toughnefs of its Pia Mater, gives more additional Support to the Lens than we might be apt to fuppofe from its general Tendernefs; it is itfelf fupported in its place, befides ferving the ufe before mentioned, of receiving Impreffions by the Light reflected from the Bottom of the Eye.

In the feveral Figures of Table Firft, and Table Firft *, thefe Parts are delineated; and to the Explanation of them I fhall refer the Reader.

CHAP.

CHAP. V.

Of the Iris.

SECT. I.

IN the Book I publiſhed on Fiſhes *, I ſtated the ſeveral circumſtances which prove, beyond doubt, that the Veſſels of the Iris are not Colourleſs, as RUYSCH, VIEUSSENS, FERREIN, Dr HALLER, ZINN, and others, following them †, have taught;

* Chap. xi.

† RUYSCH, Ep. xiii.—VIEUSSENS, Tr. de Lin. p. 211.—FERREIN, Mem. de l'Acad. (1739).—HALLER, El. Phyſ. Lib. xvi. Sect. ii. § xxxiii. p. 435. " Ex " eo porro Circulo numeroſa Vaſcula in Uveam veniunt, in variis Animalibus, " et

taught; but that, on the contrary, they are Large, Red, Numerous, and circulate an extraordinary quantity of Red Blood.

Since that time, I have obſerved, in one caſe, a White Speck on the Iris, produced by Inflammation, on the Surface of which I could ſee diſtinctly Veſſels filled with Red Blood.

In three other caſes, I have obſerved a very remarkable appearance, which, ſo far as I know, has eſcaped the obſervation of Oculiſts.

In two of theſe caſes, where the Eyes had been long inflamed, a Network of Filaments paſſed from one ſide of the Iris, acroſs the Pupil, to the other ſide of it, covered with Paint of the ſame colour with that of the Iris.

In

" et imprimis in Piſcibus, Sanguine plena, in Homine pellucida."—Zinn de Oculo, Cap. ii. p. 92. Not. *f.* " Ut inde elici poſſe videatur in Homine vivo, Vaſcula " liquorem ſanguine tenuiorem et decolorem vehere."

In the third cafe, of a Perfon who had had a White Cataract in one of his Eyes for upwards of Twenty Years, a Network of Veffels, covered with Paint darker than that of the Iris, was extended from the Iris upon the Surface of the Cataract.

I pointed out thefe appearances, in one of the cafes, to Mr ANDERSON, Surgeon in Leith, and, in another, to Mr LAW, Surgeon in Edinburgh, who were attending the Patients along with me.

SECT. II.

THE Nerves of the Iris are fo numerous, that, proportioned to its Weight, no part of the Human Body is perhaps fo plentifully fupplied with them.

SECT. III.

BUT, what account are we to give of its Muſcular Fibres; or of thoſe Fibres by means of which its motions are performed?

When we look into the Works of Dr HALLER, we find this celebrated Author, after quoting the accounts given by others, affirming, in the moſt pointed manner, That, although he examined the Iris of the Ox with the Microſcope, he could not perceive in it any Circular Fibres: And his Pupil and Succeſſor (Dr WRISBERG) affirms the ſame *.

Confiding

---

* HALLER. El. Phyſ. Lib. xvi. Sect. II. p. 371. "Ex hypotheſi, plurimi "Scriptores Fibras eſſe, in circulum circumductas. Verum eas ſæpe, et myopibus "meis, cætera bonis, oculis, et lentibus vitreis, vehementer augentibus, adjutis "cum quærerem, nunquam reperi ullas."—p. 378. "Circulus in Uvea conſtrictor "nullus eſt."——HALLER. Pr. Lin. Phyſ. § DXII. "Orbiculares Fibras, con- "centricas

Confiding in the accuracy of Dr HALLER, I, for many years, examined this organ with lefs attention than, probably, I fhould otherwife have done. But having, at laft, examined carefully the Iris of an Ox, after wafhing off the Paint, I was not more pleafed than furprifed, to find, on its Anterior Part, a broad flat oval Organ, with Fibres of a dark reddifh Colour, difpofed in nearly the fame manner as thofe of the Orbicularis Palpebrarum are.

Its appearance is, in all refpects, fo evidently Mufcular, that I think there can be no doubt of its being the Sphincter of the Pupil: And I can only account for its having efca-

O 2 ped

" centricas Pupillæ, neque Oculus, neque Microfcopium, ne in Bove quidem, mihi " demonftravit."

In a tranflation of Notes by Dr WRISBERG on HALLER's Primæ Lineæ, the Doctor writes as follows: " Befides anatomical proofs, by which it is undoubted- " ly certain, that the Iris has no real Mufcular Fibres, and that the contraction and " dilatation of the Pupil is rather to be afcribed to the Veffels than to Mufcles."

ZINN de Oculo, Cap. ii. Sect. iii. § iv. p. 91. " Dubius certe hæreo, annon " Fabrica Mufculofa in Iride agnofcenda effe videtur."

ped the obſervation of Dr HALLER and Dr WRISBERG, by ſuppoſing, that they had not waſhed off the Black Paint, which covers and conceals it, as well as the Red Veſſels of the Iris.

On the Inner and Anterior Part of the Iris, and on the whole of its Poſterior Part, the Fibres are diſpoſed like Radii; and, if they are Muſcular, they are well ſituated for dilating the Pupil. But theſe have many more Blood-veſſels in their compoſition, and have much leſs the appearance of Muſcular Fibres, than the oval fibrous Organ I have deſcribed on the Forepart of the Iris.

In Table II. Fig. 1. and 2. theſe Parts are elegantly and accurately repreſented, from Drawings made of them, at my requeſt, by Mr FYFE.

My ſucceſs in the Ox naturally prompted me to examine the Human Iris with greater attention than I had formerly beſtowed on it; and in this I found, with equal ſatisfaction, a very diſtinct Sphincter Muſcle; but ſomewhat differently diſpoſed; for in Man it occupies the Innermoſt Part of the Iris, or forms a Ring immediately ſurrounding the Pupil, which is equally well ſeen on its Fore and Back Parts, and makes

makes about One-Fifth Part of the Breadth of the Iris. Between the Sphincter and Root of the Iris, the Space is filled up with Veſſels and Radiated Fibres.

See Table III. and its Explanation.

Dr ZINN, Dr HALLER, and Dr WRISBERG *, particularly the two latter, have doubted of, or denied, the Muſcular, or, as they ſpeak, Irritable nature of the Iris; becauſe the Contraction of the Pupil is not occaſioned by Strong Light falling upon it.

But

---

* ZINN de Oculo, Cap. ii. Sect. iii. § iv. p. 95.

HALLER. El. Phyſ. Lib. xvi. Sect. ii. p. 371. "Nam, per experimenta ſolicitè "capta, Iris in vivo animale Irritabilitate omni deſtituitur, ipſiſque a lucis radiis, "per conum chartaceam in ſolam Iridem determinatis, non movetur; ſed Muſ"culo proprium eſt, eſſe irritabilem."

WRISBERG, in a Note on HALLER, Pr. Lin. Phyſ. § DXIII. "My own ex"periments have convinced me, that the Iris does not belong to the parts en"dowed with regular Irritability; for the ſolar light directed upon the Iris re"mains without any ſuch effect."

But their inference is by no means to be admitted.

Becaufe, without alleging that its being roufed into action by the irritation of the Retina, is fcarcely to be explained, but on the fuppofition that the Living Principle is firft excited, and a Mufcular Action in confequence produced; I would obferve, that the Colour or Paint upon the Iris, which prevents the Light from getting to the Bottom of the Eye except through the Pupil, muft, like a Cuticula, prevent the Light from irritating the Iris, unlefs we fuppofe it to be concentrated in a very great degree.

In the next place, we are to confider, that, in the common offices of life, Light is collected into a Focus, or fo concentrated, that it may prove hurtful to the Retina alone; and therefore Nature has, in general, regulated the action of the Iris, according to the Quantity of the Light which falls upon the Retina.

I would further obferve, that various other Mufcles are thrown into a more fudden and violent action, by Stimuli applied to diftant organs, than if the fame Stimuli had been directly applied to thofe Mufcles. Thus, if a Drop of Cold Water, or even a Drop of Warm Saliva, falls into the Glot-

tis,

tis, the very diſtant Abdominal Muſcles are ſuddenly convulſed. I ſurely need not ſay, that the Warm Saliva, directly applied to thoſe Muſcles, laid bare by diſſection, would produce no ſuch effect.

In the laſt place, I have, many years ago, obſerved in the Parrot, that the Pupil is, alternately, greatly contracted and dilated, whilſt the Eye is expoſed to the ſame degree of faint Light *; which is quite inconſiſtent with the idea, that the action of the Iris is produced by the ſole and direct effect of Stimuli applied to it.

CHAP.

* See Dr PORTERFIELD's Book on the Eyes, Vol. ii. Chap. v. p. 151.

CHAP. VI.

Of the Veſſels of the Cornea.

SECT. I.

IN the Book which I publiſhed on the Structure and Phyſiology of Fiſhes, in the year 1785, I obſerved, (Ch. XI.) that the Veſſels containing Red Blood, which are ſeen upon the Cornea after an Inflammation of it, are not its original Veſſels dilated, but are newly-formed Veſſels, rooted in the Tunica Adnata, and extended, from it, over the External Surface of the Cornea; and hence, that Surgeons might perceive the propriety of attempting to remove theſe, and the Specks produced by them, by Chirurgical means and External applications.

I would now obſerve, that, in every caſe I have examined ſince that time, I have found a confirmation of the truth of the above aſſertion.

SECT. II.

It may be worth while to add, that, on examining an Opake Circle, which, in many very old Perſons, encroaches upon the Cornea, I have found that Circle full of very minute Veſſels, rooted likewiſe in the Adnata, and extended on the External Surface of the Cornea, without entering between its Layers.

CHAP.

CHAP. VII.

Of certain Laws by which we judge of the Poſition and Diſtance of Objects, and by which we regulate the Motions of the Eyes.

SECT. I.

ALTHOUGH the whole Picture of an Object formed on the Bottom of the Eye be inverted, we form a juſt judgment of the Poſition of its Parts; becauſe we are taught by Inſtinct, that each Pencil of Rays which ſtrikes the Retina muſt have come from the oppoſite ſide. Juſt as, when our Hand is held ſupine in the horizontal poſture, if the

Back of it be ſtruck, we ſuppoſe the ſtroke to have come from Below; and, if the Palm, from Above.

I apprehend we are further taught by Inſtinct, that the Light has paſſed through the Pupil, and that we therefore form a more correct idea of the Poſition of the Object, than when, with Authors *, we imagine, that the Light is traced perpendicularly from the Place of the Picture.

SECT. II.

As we derive many advantages from directing the Axes of the Two Eyes to the ſame point, the ſuppoſition made by Authors, that this Direction is not given by Inſtinct, but proceeds

* Dr PORTERFIELD and Dr REID.——See Dr REID's Inquiry into the Human Mind, On Seeing, Chap. vi. Sect. xii. p. 261. " A viſible object appears in the " direction of a right line, perpendicular to the retina at that point where its " image is painted."

proceeds from Cuftom and Habit *, muft, at firft fight, appear extremely improbable; and the more I have attended to the Motions of the Eyes, not only in Infants, but in other very young Animals, the more I am convinced that the Uniform Motion of the Eyes, and the accurate Direction of Both to One Point, is Original.

We may obferve many other Complex Actions, Refpiration, Sucking, Deglutition, performed without Experience: Why then doubt that the Uniform Motion of the Eyes is regulated by a fimilar Law?

That, by Habit, we are lefs able to move the Eyes in different Directions in the advanced than in the early period of life, is at the fame time true.

SECT.

* Dr PORTERFIELD on the Eye, Vol. I. Book ii. Chap. v. p. 23. "The true "caufe of this uniform motion depends on Cuftom and Habit."

Dr REID, p. 240. "Nature hath very wifely left us the power of varying "the parallelifm of our Eyes a little, fo that we can direct them to the fame "point, whether remote or near. This no doubt is learned by Cuftom."

SECT. III.

The Direction of the Optic Axes furnishes, no doubt, an auxiliary means by which we judge of the Distances of Objects; but strange oversights have been committed by Authors on this subject, and particularly by Dr Porterfield, who supposes effects to proceed solely from this cause, which evidently flow from others.

Thus, he tells us, that when a Person has had the misfortune of losing one of his Eyes, or even if a Person shuts one of his Eyes, he cannot readily fill out a dish of tea, or snuff a candle, because he wants the concurrence of the Optic Axes; without considering, that the degree of action or straining of the Muscles necessary to direct the Axis of One Eye to the object, would have nearly the same effect on the Mind as the Direction of Both Axes to the same point. Besides, he forgets, that the Axis of the Eye which is shut, and even that of the blind Eye, for a long time at least, follows the motion of the other.

In

In like manner, in his principal experiment by which he proves that the Eyes accommodate themſelves to the Diſtances of Objects, he obſerves, that if we ſhut the Left Eye, and, with the Right Eye, view a Luminous Point through two ſmall Holes in a Card, this Point will appear Single at a certain diſtance to which the Eye is accommodated, but will appear Double in all other ſituations; becauſe the Rays of Light which paſs through ſmall Holes, form ſuch diſtinct Pictures, that the Eye is not ſolicited to alter its Conformation to the Diſtance. And he proves that the above is a juſt account, by next obſerving, that if the Left Eye is opened, and Both Eyes directed to the Luminous Point, the Double appearance of it inſtantly vaniſhes. But, in attempting to explain the Cauſes which prompt the Mind to act, he ſuppoſes, that the Two Optic Axes being now directed to the ſame Point, we are enabled to take the Angle, and ſo meaſure the Diſtance; not reflecting, that the Axis of the Left Eye, whilſt it was Shut, was guided by the Direction of the Open Eye, or had had the ſame Direction when it was Shut, as when it was Opened.

Hence Dr PORTERFIELD, though he proves, by this experiment, that the Eye alters its Conformation, has not pointed ed out the true Means by which it judges of the Diſtance, and is therefore ſolicited to act.

Theſe, I apprehend, in this caſe, depend on the clearer view which the Two Eyes receive, not only of the Luminous Point, but of the relative Situation of the ſeveral Objects which are nearer to or farther from us than it; by means of which the Mind judges more accurately of the Diſtance, and therefore accommodates the Eye to it.

CHAP.

CHAP. VIII.

Of the Means by which we accommodate the Eye to the Diſtances of Objects.

THAT the Human Eye poſſeſſes the power of accommodating itſelf to the Diſtances of Objects, ſeems beyond a doubt *: And, I think, I can prove, that this power is not reſtricted within the narrow limit of Twenty-ſeven Inches, as Dr PORTERFIELD contends; for I find, that when I place two minute Objects in nearly the ſame line, the neareſt of them at the diſtance of Three Feet, and the other at double or treble that diſtance, on viewing them alternately with one Eye, they become alternately confuſed and diſtinct.

* See Dr PORTERFIELD on the Eyes.

But, to aſcertain the Means by which the Eye accommodates itſelf to the Diſtances of Objects, is a matter of much difficulty.

The following are the chief Means enumerated; on each of which I ſhall make a few Remarks. And I ſhall then point out an Additional Means, which has eſcaped the obſervation of Authors.

SECT. I.

It has been ſuppoſed, that the Fibres which enter into the compoſition of the Cryſtalline Lens are Muſcular, and that, by their Contraction, they render the Lens more Convex, and therefore adapt the Eye to near Objects. But to this opinion I have, in the First Chapter of this Paper, propoſed Objections, to which I ſhall refer the Reader.

SECT.

SECT. II.

THE Ciliary Proceſſes have been ſuppoſed to be chief agents. But, without ſtating, that Muſcular Fibres are not to be ſeen in theſe Proceſſes *, or the improbability that the Choroid Coat, of which they are the Continuation, in the form of Folds or Doublings, is Muſcular, as its general action would be uſeleſs and even injurious to the Retina; and without repeating the argument, that the Eye ſeems to accommodate itſelf after the Extraction of the Lens;—I would remind the Reader, that their Extremities float looſe in the Aqueous Humour, and that their Inner-part is connected to the Lens by the medium of the Retina: Nor is their direction ſuch, that they can be ſuppoſed capable of pulling the Lens forwards, by pulling the Retina: Or, if we were to ſuppoſe them to be Muſcular, and to act with conſiderable force, they would render the Lens flatter, by pulling its

 Circular

* ZINN, Cap. ii. p. 70. "Neque unquam Microſcopio unicam Fibram Muſcu-"larem reperiri potui."

Circular Edge outwards, and would therefore have the effect, contrary to what is ſuppoſed, of rendering the Eye leſs fit for viewing near objects.

SECT. III.

THE Iris, by leſſening the Pupil, and cutting off the moſt diverging rays of light, when we are viewing near objects, unqueſtionably makes the Picture on the Retina more diſtinct, and therefore renders the Object more diſtinct.

SECT. IV.

SOME, as JURIN, have thought, that the Iris might, by its Contraction, have the effect of drawing the Root of the Cornea inwards; and, by this means, render the Cornea more Convex: And the Diſpoſition of the Sphincter Muſcle of the Iris, eſpecially in the Ox, may ſeem to ſupport this opinion.

But

But I muſt obſerve, That the Iris is not Rooted in the Cornea, as thoſe who maintain this opinion ſuppoſe, but in the Sclerotic Coat, which in Man is thicker and reſiſts more than the Cornea, and in many other Animals is remarkably hard and inflexible. Beſides this, I have ſhewn, that, in Man, the Sphincter Muſcle of the Iris is placed on the Inner Edge of the Iris, with the interpoſition of the Radiated Vaſcular Subſtance between it and the Sclerotic; ſo that it cannot directly affect the Sclerotic and Cornea.

To theſe we may add, that, in a clear light, when the Iris is ſtrongly contracted, we ſee remote objects diſtinctly: Whereas, if the ſtrong contraction of the Iris which then takes place, rendered the Cornea more Convex, and thereby fitted the Eye for near objects, thoſe ſhould appear confuſed.

SECT. V.

The External Muſcles, and particularly the Recti, have, by many, been thought to be well adapted for elongating the Axis of the Eye; and a late Writer alleges, that the

Recti.

Recti terminate partly in the External Layer of the Cornea, and therefore are better ſuited, than was imagined, for ſuch a purpoſe. But here I would obſerve, in the firſt place, That, on re-examining this point of Anatomy with attention, I have found all the Tendinous Fibres of the Recti firmly attached to the Sclerotic, at the diſtance of a quarter of an inch from the Edge of the Cornea, and no appearance that any part of them, or that any Membrane produced by them, is continued over the Cornea *.

In

---

* By experiment on the Human Eye, I found, that the Weight of Fifty-four Ounces tore one of the Recti Muſcles; but that it required the Weight of a Hundred Ounces to tear its Tendon from the Sclerotic Coat, and when the Tendon quitted the Sclerotic, there was no appearance ſeen of its Fibres paſſing forwards over the Cornea. And, the generally very accurate, ZINN, who had no particular Theory to ſupport or to refute, expreſſes himſelf on this ſubject in the following words: " Tendines illorum Muſculorum ſinguli, etſi ad inſertionem latiores evadunt, diſtincti tamen ſemper manent, et, ubi immiſſis in Scleroticam " Fibris, illi tam intimè jam affiguntur, ut ſine manifeſta laceratione ulteriùs dividi " non poſſint, ſatis magno inter ſe diſtant intervallo, nec alibi ſeſe contingunt, ut, " nunquam in unum jungi, aut propriam tunicam continuam conſtituere poſſe, affirmari poſſit." ZINN de Oculo, Cap. i. p. 14.

In the next place, if they had terminated partly in the External Layer of the Cornea, in ſuch a manner as to affect it chiefly, they ſhould, by pulling the whole External Layer of the Cornea backwards, have flattened the Cornea, inſtead of rendering it more convex.

SECT. VI.

About fifteen years ago, it occurred to me, that, although we ſhould grant, to Dr Porterfield and others, that the Axis of the Eye could not be elongated by the Recti Muſcles; yet, that the Oblique Muſcles, which are thrown, in oppoſite directions, around the Eyeball, might have this effect. I have ſince obſerved, that Dr Keil, Hambergerus, and other Phyſiologiſts, had long ago entertained the ſame idea *.

To

* Dr Keil, Ang. Chap. iv. Sect. iv. "The Aqueous Humour, being the "thinneſt and moſt liquid, eaſily changes its figure, when either the Ligamentum "Ciliare

To be better underftood, I had a Preparation and Drawing made of the Oblique Mufcles; from which Table III. was engraved.

SECT. VII.

I SHALL conclude, by pointing out one other Means, that had not occurred to Authors, which we employ when we view minute objects placed near to the Eyes.

If we attend to what paffes in that cafe, we may be fenfible that we bring the Upper and Under Eyelids nearer to each other; and then, by a confiderable exertion, contract the parts about the Eyes.

On

" Ciliare contracts, or both the Oblique Mufcles fqueeze the middle of the Bulb of " the Eye, to render it oblong, when objects are too near us." —— BRIGGS et HAMBERGER. de Oculo, p. 180. propofe the fame opinion.

On confidering this, it appeared to me probable, that the Orbicular Mufcle of the Eyelids might, by its preffure on the Upper and Under Parts of the Cornea, make thefe fomewhat Flatter, and, of courfe, protrude the Middle Part of the Cornea between the Edges of the Eyelids, fo as to render it more Convex; at the fame time increafing its diftance from the Lens, and lengthening the Axis of the Eyeball.

On putting this matter to the teft of the following Experiments, the event appeared to correfpond exactly with the idea I had formed.

EXPERIMENT I.

In a clofet, lighted by a fingle window, I fat on a chair, with my back to the window, and fixed a Book, with Small Print, on the oppofite wall. I then brought my Eyes fo near to the Book, that the Letters became indiftinct. I then made an Exertion to read, without contracting the Orbicularis; or, I opened the Eyelids wide, by acting with the Attollens Palpebram Superiorem; or, I held the Upper and Under Eyelids with my fingers at a diſtance from each other, and then repeated my effort to read the Book; but found I could not do it. That is, my Eyes were ſo near to the Book, that, although I attempted to exert all the means before enumerated, the Eyes were not ſo much altered in their conformation as to render the viſion diſtinct. In this Experiment, no part of the Cornea was covered by the Eyelids, for the Eyelids were at the diſtance of Half an Inch from each other.

EXPERIMENT II.

In this Experiment, I kept my head in the ſame poſture, and at the ſame diſtance from the Book, as in the former Experiment; but I acted with the Orbicularis Palpebrarum, ſo as to bring the Edges of the Eyelids within a Quarter of an Inch of each other, and then made an exertion to read, and found I could ſee the Letters and Words diſtinctly.

EX-

EXPERIMENT III.

In this Experiment, I kept my head in the ſame poſture, and at the ſame diſtance from the Book, as in the two former Experiments; but, inſtead of employing the Muſcular Contraction of the Orbicularis Palpebrarum, I brought the Edges of the Upper and Under Eyelids within a Quarter of an Inch of each other, by means of my fingers, and then ſtretched the Edges of the Eyelids ſo as to make Preſſure on the Upper and Under Edges of the Cornea; and found that the Letters then appeared diſtinct.

As, in all theſe Experiments, the Diſtance of the Eye from the Object, and the Quantity of Light, were the ſame; as no Part of the Pupil was covered by the Eyelids, ſo as to cut off the moſt diverging Rays; as the Object appeared confuſed when the Orbicularis was not contracted; and diſtinct on its contracting; — there can be no doubt that the Action of the Orbicularis helps to accommodate the Eye for seeing near Objects more distinctly *.

SECT.

---

* On the 1st day of May 1794, Dr DAVID HOSACK read to the Royal Society of London, Observations on Vision, in which (Phil. Trans. 1794, Part. II. xv. p. 222.) he writes as follows: "With a Speculum, I made pressure on the Eye, "while directing attention to an Object twenty yards distant, and saw it distinctly: "but, endeavouring to look beyond it, every thing appeared confused.

"I then increased the Pressure considerably, in consequence of which I was "enabled to see objects distinctly at a much nearer than the natural focal distance; "for example, I held a Book before my Eye at the distance of two inches. In "the natural state of the Eye, I could neither distinguish Lines nor Letters: but, "on making Pressure with the Speculum, I was enabled to distinguish both Lines "and Letters of the Book with ease."

I find myself, therefore, under the disagreeable necessity of adding, That I mentioned the above Experiments, in my Public Course of Lectures, on the 27th day of April 1789:—That I have repeated the mention of them in every Course of my Lectures since that time:—That Dr WHEATON BRADISH, in his Inaugural Dissertation "De Visu," published on September 12. 1792, and which I did not read till it was published, mentions, in p. 39. these opinions, which I had proposed in my Lectures, in the following words: "Longè verò ante alias enitescit sententia, quæ interni auxilio cujusvis spreto, Musculos quosdam Oculi externos, obliquos nempè, insuper et Orbicularem, hos simul præstare effectus asseruit. Tali modo "Oculi

SECT. VIII.

Upon the whole: it appears to me,

1. That the Iris, by leſſening the Pupil, and intercepting the moſt diverging Rays of Light, renders the Picture of near Objects more diſtinct.

2. That the Recti Muſcles, by their action, lengthen the Axis, becauſe they preſs chiefly on the Sides of the Eyeball; and, further, the Cornea is not only more dilatable than the Sclerotic in general is, but it will be found that the Sclerotic, in Man and other Animals, is thinner and more dilatable, in its Anterior Part, and in its Poſterior Part where the Picture is formed, than it is on its Sides.

3. That

" Oculi Axin augeri, Corneamque convexam magis quam antea reddi."—That Dr DAVID HOSACK attended my Courſe of Lectures the winter after Dr BRADISH publiſhed his Inaugural Diſſertation, to wit, 1792–3, which was finiſhed upwards of a year before Dr HOSACK read his Paper to the Royal Society.

3. That the two Oblique Mufcles forming an Oblique Girth around the Eyeball, between the Lens and Bottom of the Eye, muft, by their Preffure, increafe the Diftance of the Lens from the Retina, or increafe the Length of the Pofterior Part of the Axis of the Eyeball.

4. The Orbicularis Palpebrarum renders the Fore and Middle Part of the Cornea, oppofite to the Pupil, more Convex; and increafes the Length of the Anterior Part of the Axis of the Eyeball. And it is evident that all thefe Means may concur in forming perfect Vifion.

CHAP.

CHAP. IX.

Of the Lachrymal Ducts.

SECT. I.

VERY eminent Authors, HALLER and ZINN, having ſtarted their doubts of the Exiſtence of Ducts from the Glandula Innominata of GALEN *, I was led to examine the ſubject

* HALLER, in Pr. Lin. Phyſ. Cap. xviii. § 498. "Lachrymam partim arteriæ conjunctivæ tunicæ exhalant, partim creditur deponere Glandula," &c. "In Homine nondum ſatis certo, neque mihi unquám viſi ſunt Ductus."

T. G. ZINN,

ſubject with accuracy; and, after finding one large Duct from it in Birds, I diſcovered a number of ſmall Ducts from it in the Human Body, running nearly parallel with each other, and terminating on the Inner-ſide of the Upper Eye-lid, not far from the External Canthus of the Eye.

After introducing Briſtles into ſome of them, I injected Quickſilver into a few others; and I ſtill preſerve the Preparations I made then, and have demonſtrated them, ſince that time, annually in my Public Courſes of Lectures. In 1758, I publiſhed a Deſcription of them *, illuſtrated by the Figures reprinted in Table IV. of this Paper.

SECT.

T. G. ZINN, de Oculo, Cap. xiii. § 1. "Lachrymas maxima certè ex parte "exhalare videtur arteriæ conjunctivæ," &c. "In Homine autem huc uſque "accuratiſſimorum Anatomicorum aciem Ductus illi effugerunt: neque mihi, hac "in re, illis feliciorem eſſe contigit."

* Obſervations Anatomical and Phyſiological, 1758, 8vo.

SECT. II.

SINCE that time, finding that the error had been committed, by the greater number of Anatomifts and Surgeons, of fuppofing, that the Two Ducts which lead from the Puncta are united before they enter the Lachrymal Sac; and thinking, that, in certain cafes, it might be material in the cure, that the Surgeon knew that one of thefe Ducts might be pervious, though the other was obftructed; I had an accurate Drawing of them, and of the Lachrymal Sac, and Nafal Duct, made, which the Reader will find in Table V. Fig. 1. And, in Fig. 2. and 3. of the fame Table, the appearance of the Termination of the Nafal Duct is delineated.

SECT. III.

To trace fully the courfe of the Tears, Two other Canals, I apprehend, remain to be defcribed; I mean the Ductus Incifivi. In Quadrupeds, as in the Ox and Sheep, thefe are

Two Large Canals, open at both ends, and paſſing obliquely downwards from the Noſe into the Mouth, repreſented in Tables VI. and VII.

In by far the greater number of Human Subjects, of different ages, I have not been able to find any veſtige of ſuch Ducts, in the Bottom of the Noſe, or Roof of the Mouth: But, in a few ſubjects, I have found them, open at both ends, but always very much ſmaller than in the Quadruped. In ſome of theſe, I paſſed a Briſtle or Small Probe, very readily, from the Noſe into the Mouth. In two or three ſubjects, I firſt poured Quickſilver from the Noſe, through the Ductus Inciſivus, into the Mouth; and then, with a ſmall Syringe, injected through it Melted Wax, coloured with Vermilion: And theſe Preparations, which I have preſerved and demonſtrated for a great number of years, are accurately delineated in Table V. Fig. 4, 5, 6, 7.

SECT. IV.

In Man, and in the Quadruped, the Lachrymal Ducts are always directed towards the Forepart of the Noſe, and terminate

minate over the Ductus Incisivi; and the Ductus Incisivi begin from Cups or Funnels, which form the Lowermost Parts of the Bottom of the Nostrils: So that, beyond all doubt, the Tears are applied to and pass through them into the mouth; and it seems by no means improbable, that the Ductus Incisivi, like the Puncta Lachrymalia and Ducts through which the Tears are conveyed into the Nose, may be excited into action by that kind of Irritation which the Tears give. Why they are always found, and large, in the Quadruped; yet generally wanting, and always small, in Man; cannot, without farther observation, be satisfactorily explained.

TAB. I.

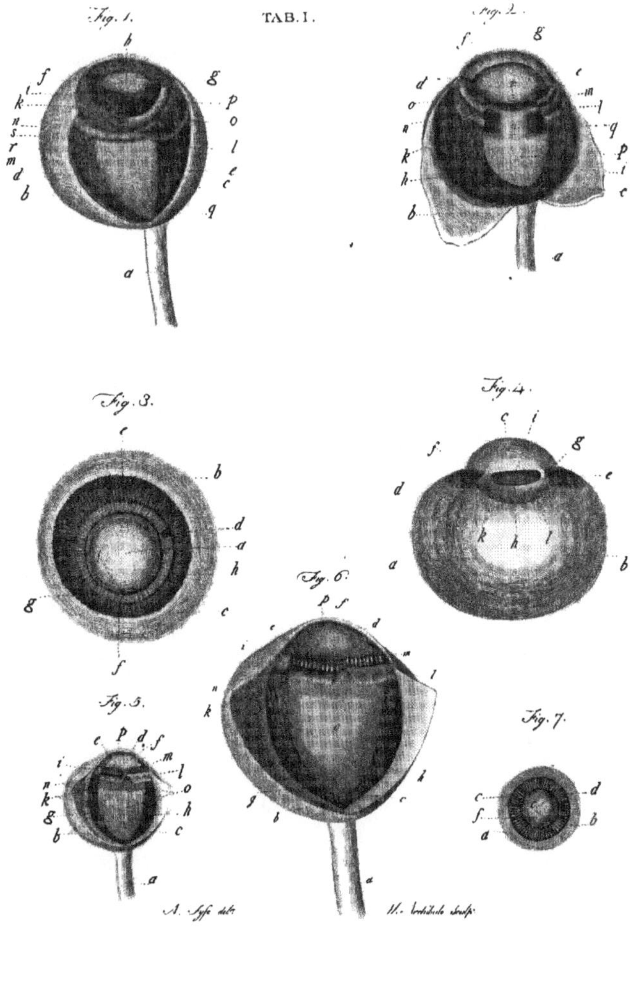

EXPLANATION

OF THE

T A B L E S.

Explanation of Table I.

THE First Four Figures of this Table represent the Eye of an Ox dissected. The Fifth, Sixth, and Seventh Figures represent the Human Eye.

FIG.

FIG. 1.

Reprefents the Left Eye of an Ox, viewed obliquely from above.

a The Trunk of the Optic Nerve.

b c The Outer Part of the Sclerotic Coat.

d e The Cut Edge of the Sclerotic Coat.

f g A Section of the Root of the Cornea.

h The Cryftalline Lens, feen at the Pupil, inclofed in its Capfule.

i The Inner Radiated Part of the Iris.

k The Sphincter Mufcle of the Iris.

l m The Outer-fide of the Choroid Coat.

n The

n The Ciliary Circle, joining the Choroid Coat to the Root of the Iris, and Both theſe Coats to the Sclerotic Coat.

o A Portion of the Iris inverted, after cutting it.

p The Ciliary Proceſſes of the Choroid Coat, the Extremities of which float in the Poſterior Chamber of the Aqueous Humour, or between the Back-part of the Iris and the Cryſtalline Lens.

q The Retina iſſuing from the Optic Nerve.

r The Middle Part of the Retina.

ſ The Choroid Coat, lined with its Black Paint, between the Ciliary Circle and the Continuation of the Retina forwards.

In

In FIG. 2.

The ſame Eye is repreſented more fully diſſected.

a Repreſents the Trunk of the Optic Nerve.

b c The Sclerotic Coat cut and turned aſide.

d e A Section of the Cornea near its Root.

f The Under Half of the Iris.

g The Cryſtalline Lens incloſed in its Capſule.

h i The Outer-ſide of the Choroid Coat.

k l The Ciliary Circle.

m The Ciliary Proceſſes, with their Extremities floating in the Aqueous Humour between the Iris and the Lens.

n A

n A Portion of the Iris inverted.

o The Extremities of a Number of the Ciliary Proceſſes inverted, to ſhew how far they are looſe.

p The Middle Part of the Retina.

q The Doublings or Ciliary Proceſſes of the Retina, from which the Black Paint, lining the Ciliary Proceſſes of the Choroid Coat, is waſhed off.

r The Ciliary Proceſſes of the Retina divided into Minute Fibres, which are inſerted into the Anterior Part of the Capſule of the Cryſtalline Lens.

In FIG. 3.

After removing the Cornea, the Iris, the Choroid Coat with its Paint, and inflating the Canal difcovered by Dr PETIT, a Fore View is given of the Cryftalline Lens, with the Termination of the Retina, by Doublings or Ciliary Proceffes, in the Forepart of the Capfule of the Lens, a very little within its Outer Edge.

a Reprefents the Forepart of the Cryftalline inclofed in its Capfule.

b c The Vitreous Humour covered by the Retina.

d A Hole cut in the Forepart of the Canal of PETIT, by which it was inflated.

e f The Circular Canal of PETIT inflated, to fhew that it is not Cylindrical, but Cellular, fomewhat refembling the Colon.

g h The

g h The Doublings or Ciliary Proceſſes of the Retina, adhering to the Anterior Layer of the Capſule of the Vitreous Humour, and, with that, forming the Forepart of the Canal of PETIT.

i The Minute Terminations of the Ciliary Proceſſes of the Retina, in the Anterior Part of the Capſule of the Lens, very near to the Outer Edge of the Lens.

FIG. 4.

In this Figure, a Side View is given of the Cryſtalline Lens and Vitreous Humour adhering together, and their Capſules entire.

a b The Vitreous Humour incloſed in its Capſule.

c The Forepart of the Cryſtalline Lens.

d e The Roots of the Ciliary Proceſſes of the Retina, with ſome of the Black Paint of the Choroid Coat adhering to their Outer Side, and the Anterior Layer of the Capſule of the Vitreous Humour lining them.

f g The Inſertion of the Retina, with the Anterior Layer of the Vitreous Humour, in the Forepart of the Capſule of the Lens.

h An Oblong Hole cut in the Outer Part of the Canal of PETIT, through which the Outer Edge of the Lens is ſeen, covered with its proper Capſule, forming the Inner-ſide of the Canal of PETIT.

i The Anterior, and *k* the Poſterior, Layer of the Capſule of the Vitreous Humour, fixed to the Capſule of the Lens at a conſiderable diſtance from each other. Hence it appears, that the Forepart of the Canal of PETIT is formed by the Anterior Layer of the Vitreous Humour, covered by the Retina; the Poſterior Part of it, by the Vitreous Humour, covered by the Poſterior Layer of its Capſule;

Capſule; and that the Inner-ſide of it, is formed by the Edge of the Cryſtalline, covered by its proper Capſule only, where its greateſt Diameter is found, or where the Two Lenſes which compoſe it are conjoined.

l The Backpart of the Cryſtalline Lens ſeen through the Vitreous Humour.

FIG. 5. & 6.

In theſe Figures, the Connexion of the Coats of the Human Eye is repreſented. In Fig. 5. the Parts are repreſented of their Natural Size: In Fig. 6. they are magnified to Two Diameters.

a The Optic Nerve.

b c The Sclerotic Coat, cut and turned aſide.

d The Cut Edge of the Cornea.

e The

e The Iris.

f The Forepart of the Lens.

g h The Outer Sides of the Choroid Coat.

i The Ciliary Circle.

k l The Iris cut and turned backwards.

m The Ciliary Proceſſes of the Choroid Coat in their natural ſituation, with their Extremities floating looſe in the Aqueous Humour, and covering the Outer Edge of the Lens.

n The Extremities of the Ciliary Proceſſes turned back, to ſhew how much of them is looſe, or unconnected with the Parts on the Inner-ſide of them.

o The Middle Part of the Retina.

q The Anterior Part of the Retina, connected to the Capſule of the Lens by the Fibrous Extremities of its Ciliary Proceſſes.

FIG.

FIG. 7.

This Figure reprefents the Retina lining the Pofterior Part of the Ciliary Proceffes, and inferted into the Capfule of the Lens.

a b The Inner-fide of a Part of the Sclerotic Coat.

c d The Ciliary Proceffes of the Retina, on the Inner-fide of the Paint which lines the Ciliary Proceffes of the Choroid Coat.

f The Pofterior Part of the Cryftalline Lens inclofed in its Capfule.

e The Fibrous Extremities of the Ciliary Proceffes of the Retina, in their courfe, over the Edge of the Cryftalline Lens, to their Terminations in the Forepart of its Capfule.

Explanation

Explanation of Table I.*

FIG. 1.

Repreſents the Human Eye diſſected.

a The Optic Nerve.

b b The Sclerotic Coat, cut and turned outwards.

c The Sclerotic Coat, cut and turned forwards with the Cornea *d*.

e e One-half of the Iris in its place.

f The

TAB. I. *.

Fig. 1.

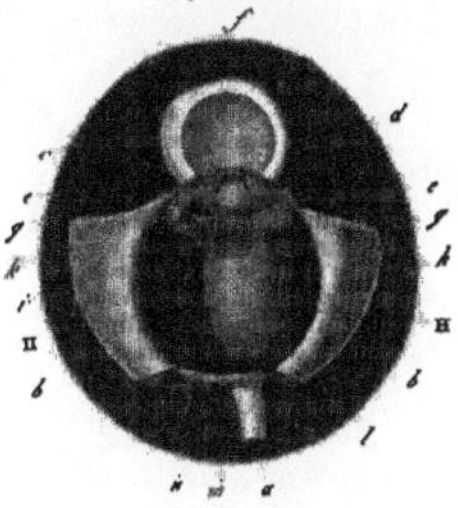

Fig. 2.

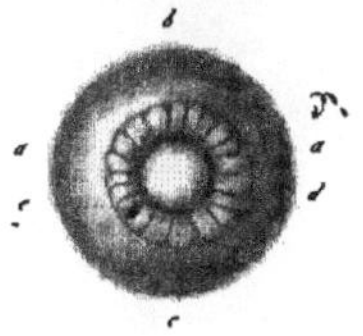

f The Pupil and Cryſtalline Lens in its place.

g g The Ciliary Circle.

H H The Choroid Coat.

h The Ciliary Proceſſes ſeen in their places, by cutting off a portion of the Iris.

i A Portion of the Iris cut and turned back.

k The Floating Points of the Ciliary Proceſſes turned backwards.

l The Middle Smooth Part of the Retina, ſeen by cutting a Hole in the Choroid Coat.

m The Roots of the Ciliary Proceſſes of the Retina, to which the Black Paint of the Ciliary Proceſſes of the Choroid Coat adheres.

n The Ciliary Proceſſes of the Retina, inſerted into the Capſule of the Cryſtalline Lens.

FIG. 2.

Reprefents, chiefly, the Circle of PETIT in the Human Eye.

a a The Vitreous Humour inclofed in its Capfule.

b The Cryftalline Lens inclofed in its Capfule.

c The Ciliary Proceffes of the Retina inferted into the Capfule of the Cryftalline Lens.

d The Circular Canal of PETIT inflated.

e A Hole cut in the Circular Canal of PETIT, at which the Air diftending it was blown in.

Explanation

TAB. II.

Fig. 1.

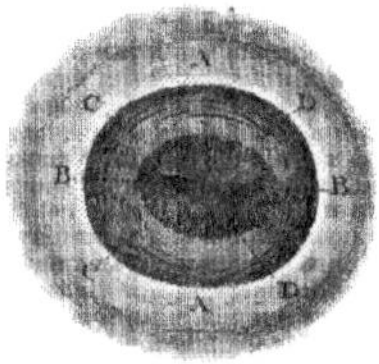

Fig. 2.

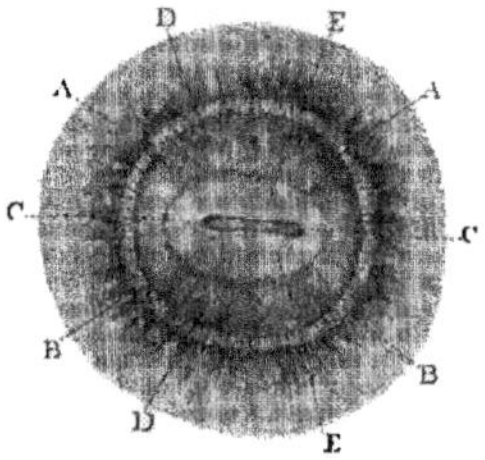

Explanation of Table II.

FIG. 1. reprefents the Forepart, and Fig. 2. the Backpart, of the Iris of an Ox, of its Natural Size.

In FIG. 1.

A A Reprefents the Cut Edge of the Sclerotic Coat.

B B The Pupil.

C C The Sphincter Mufcle of the Iris.

D D The Inner Part of the Iris, in which the Fibres are radiated, without any appearance of a Sphincter Mufcle.

In FIG. 2.

A A Repreſents the Inner-ſide of the Anterior Part of the Choroid Coat.

B B The Ciliary Proceſſes.

C C The Pupil.

D D The Outer and Back Part of the Iris, which conſiſts of Vaſcular and Radiated Fibres that conceal the Sphincter Muſcle.

E E The Inner and Back Part of the Iris, compoſed, like its Forepart, of Radiated and Vaſcular Fibres.

Explanation

TAB. III.

Fig. 1.

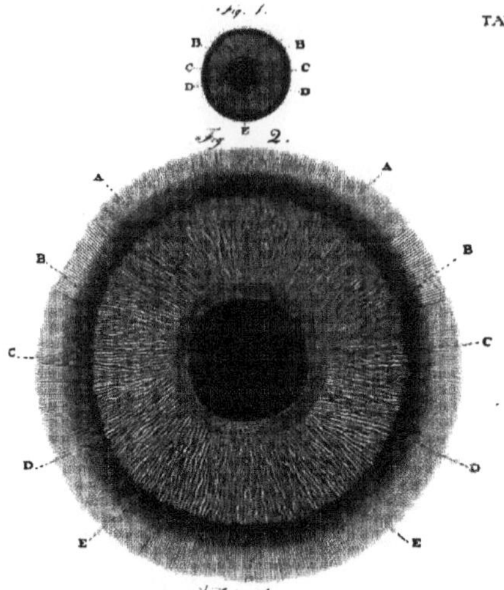

A. Fyfe del.

W. Archibald sc.

Explanation of Table III.

THE Two Figures in this Table reprefent the Pofterior Part of the Human Iris, delineated by Mr FYFE. Fig. 1. fhews it of the Natural Size, and Fig. 2. reprefents it Magnified.

A A The Inner-fide of the Anterior Part of the Choroid Coat.

B B The Ciliary Proceffes.

C C The Veffels and Radiated Fibres.

D D The Mufcular Sphincter of the Iris.

E The Pupil.

Explanation

Explanation of Table IV.

THIS Table reprefents the Right Eye with its Mufcles, viewed obliquely from its Upper and Outer Side.

a Reprefents the Eyeball.

b Part of the Upper Eyelid.

c The Optic Nerve.

d The Attollens Palpebram Superiorem drawn afide by a Pin.

e The Rectus Attollens Oculum.

f The Rectus Abductor Oculi.

g The

TAB. IV.

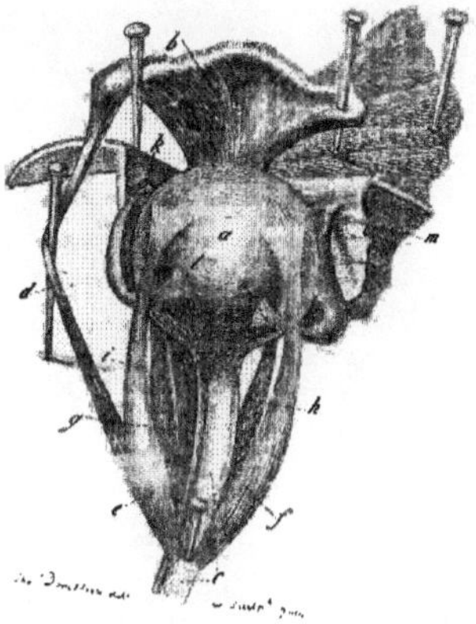

g The Rectus Adductor Oculi.

h The Rectus Deprimens Oculum.

i The Flesby Belly of the Obliquus Superior Trochlearis.

k The Trochlea, fixed to the Os Frontis, with the Tendon passing through it.

l The Insertion of the Tendon of the Trochlearis in the Eyeball.

m The Inferior Oblique Muscle taking its rise from the Superior Maxillary Bone.

n The Insertion of the Tendon of the Inferior Oblique Muscle in the Eyeball.

Explanation

Explanation of Table V.

FIG. 1.

Repreſents the Upper Eyelid of the Right Side of the Human Subject, with the Glandula Innominata GALENI, or Lachrymal Gland.

a The Inner-ſide of the Upper Eyelid.

p The Two Puncta Lachrymalia, into which the different Ends of a Bit of Wire are introduced.

b Part of the Under Eyelid.

c The External Canthus.

d The Thicker Conglomerated Part of the Lachrymal Gland.

TAB.V.

Fig. I.

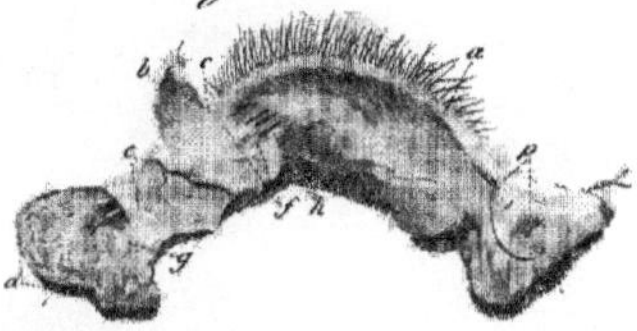

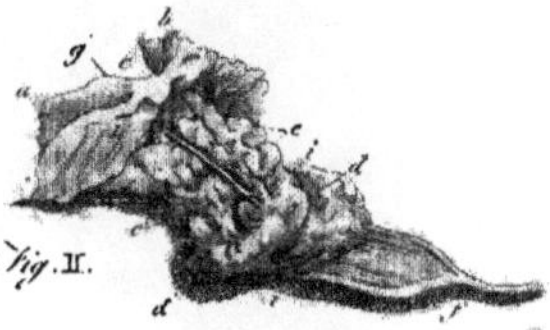

Fig. II.

Fig. III.

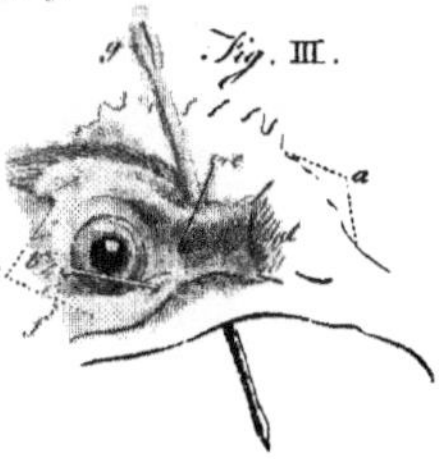

Fig. IV.

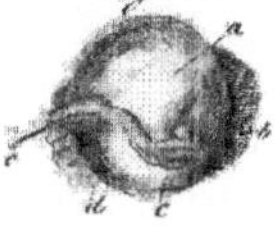

A. Bell Sculp.

e A Number of Smaller Lachrymal Glands, lying between *d* and the Conjunctiva, which, for distinction's sake, I shall call Glandulæ Lachrymales Congregatæ.

f Four Bristles introduced into the Ducts of the Lachrymal Gland.

g One of these Ducts, into which Quicksilver was injected, which is hid where it passes between the Glandulæ Congregatæ *e*, but appears again, where it comes out of the Glandula Innominata, composed of Three Branches.

h A Part of the Tunica Conjunctiva, at which, before the Preparation was immersed in Spirits, the Orifices of two or three very small Lachrymal Ducts could be perceived.

FIG. 2.

Reprefents the like Parts on the Left Side, viewed from the Upper and Outer Side.

a The Outer Side of the Tunica Conjunctiva of the Left Eye.

b c dd ee The fame as in Fig. 1.

f The Artery of the Lachrymal Gland injected.

g The End of a Briftle put into one of the Lachrymal Ducts *h*, after I had injected the Duct with Quickfilver.

i i Two Branches joining to compofe the Duct *h*.

FIG.

FIG. 3.

Repreſents the Right Eye of the Common Hen.

a An Outline of the Comb and Beak.

b The Eyeball.

c The Eyelids.

d The Membrana Nictitans.

e A Probe paſſed into the Duct of the Lachrymal Gland.

f A Probe paſſed into the Undermoſt Punctum Lachrymale.

g A Probe paſſed from the Uppermoſt Punctum Lachrymale into the Noſe, and from the Noſe into the Mouth.

In FIG. 4.

a Repreſents the Bottom of the Eyeball in the ſame Fowl.

b The Optic Nerve.

c The Lachrymal Gland.

d Part of the Membrana Nictitans.

e A Probe paſſed into the Lachrymal Duct.

Explanation

TAB.VI.

Fig. 1.

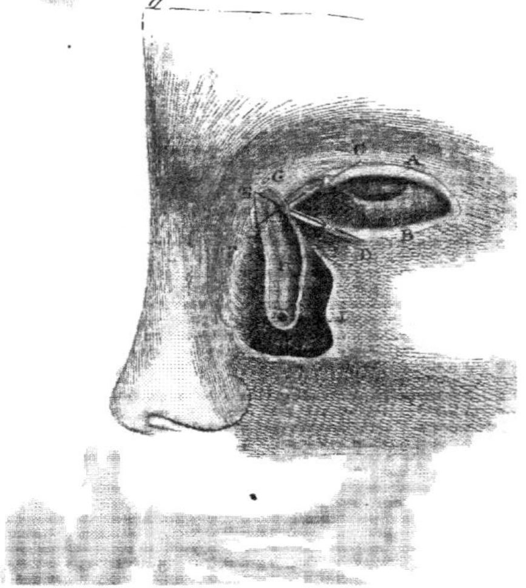

Fig. 2.

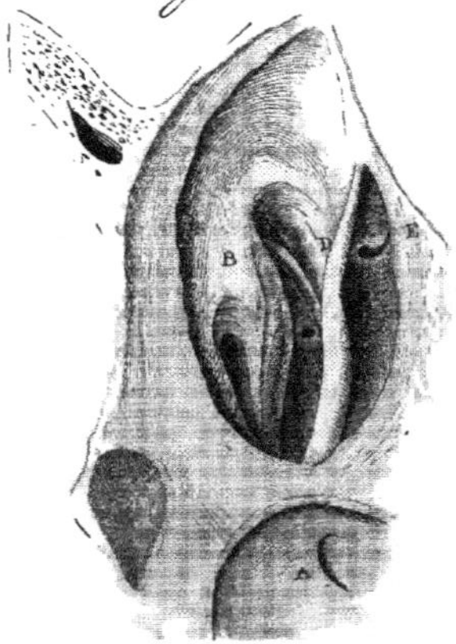

Fig. 3.

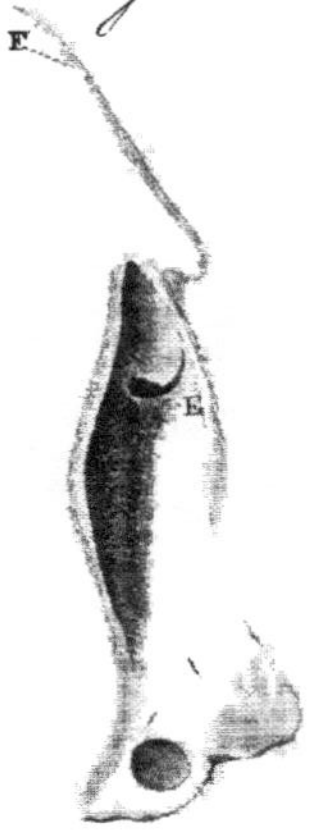

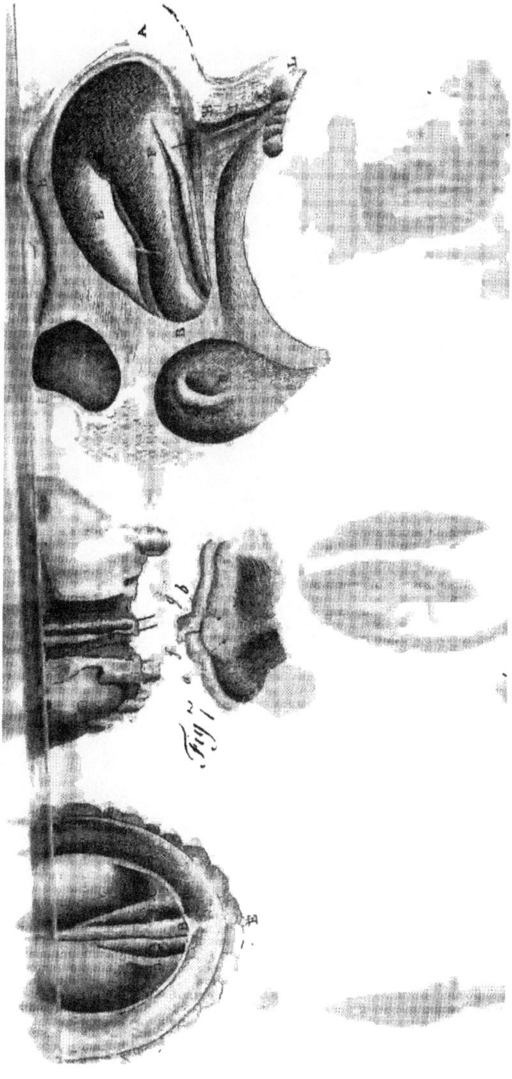

Explanation of Table VI.

In FIG. 1.

A Repreſents the Upper and B the Under Eyelid.

C D Briſtles introduced into the Two Puncta Lachrymalia, and the Ducts from them cut open.

E F The Termination of theſe Ducts in the Lachrymal Sac, by two diſtinct Orifices.

G H I The Lachrymal Sac and Naſal Duct laid open.

In

In FIG. 2. & 3.

The Termination of the Nasal Lachrymal Duct in the Nose is seen at E E, under the Os Spongiosum Inferius D.

FIG. 4.

ABBC Represents Part of the Septum Narium.

D The Mouth of the Left Eustachian Tube.

E The Superior, and F the Inferior, Os Spongiosum of the Left Side.

HIK The Ductus Incisivus of the Right Side laid open, after passing a Bristle through it.

FIG.

F I G. 5.

A B Repreſents the Septum Narium cut horizontally.

C D The Upper Orifices of the Ductus Inciſivi.

E The Dentes Inciſivi.

F I G. 6.

By cutting off the Foreparts of the Upper Jaw-Bones, the Ductus Inciſivi are ſeen, with Probes paſſed through them from the Bottom of the Noſe into the Mouth.

A The Bottom of the Septum Narium cut horizontally.

B C The Bottom of the Cavity of the Noſe.

de & *fg* Briſtles paſſed through the Ductus Inciſivi.

F I G.

FIG. 7.

In this Figure, the Openings of the Ductus Incisivi into the Mouth are represented, from a Person, very far advanced in life, who had lost all the Teeth of both Jaws.

a b The Lower Orifices of the Ductus Incisivi.

Explanation

TAB. VII.

Fig. 2.

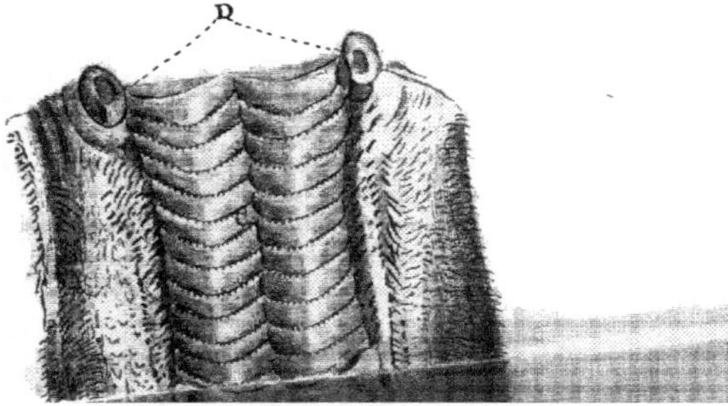

Fig. 1.

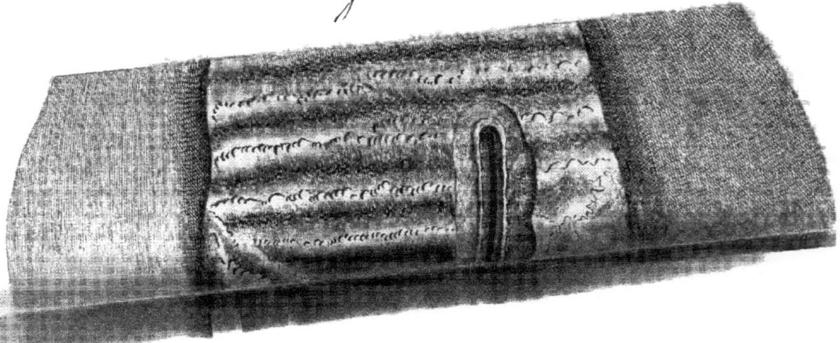

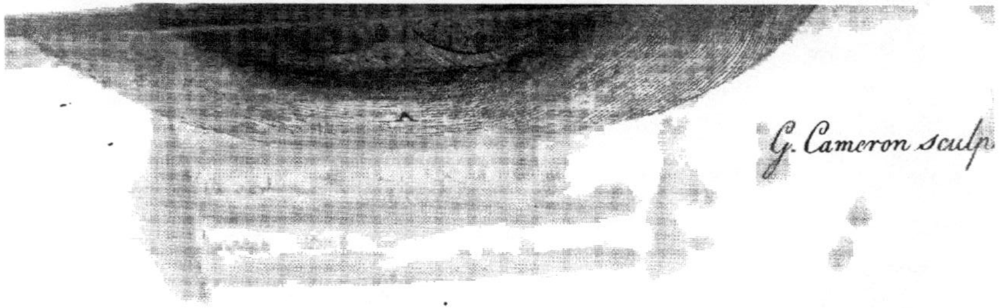

G. Cameron sculp.

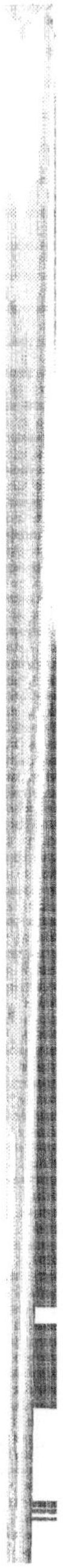

Explanation of Table VII.

FIG. 1.

A Reprefents the Upper-Lip of the Ox.

B The Callous Gum.

C The Roof of the Mouth.

E E The Natural Openings of the Two Ductus Incifivi.

F The Under Part of the Right Ductus Incifivus cut open its whole length.

In FIG. 2.

A Repreſents the Upper Lip of the Sheep.

B The Callous Gum.

C The Roof of the Mouth.

E The Natural Termination of the Left Ductus Inciſivus.

F A Probe paſſed from the Noſe, through the Right Ductus Inciſivus, into the Mouth.

TAB. VIII

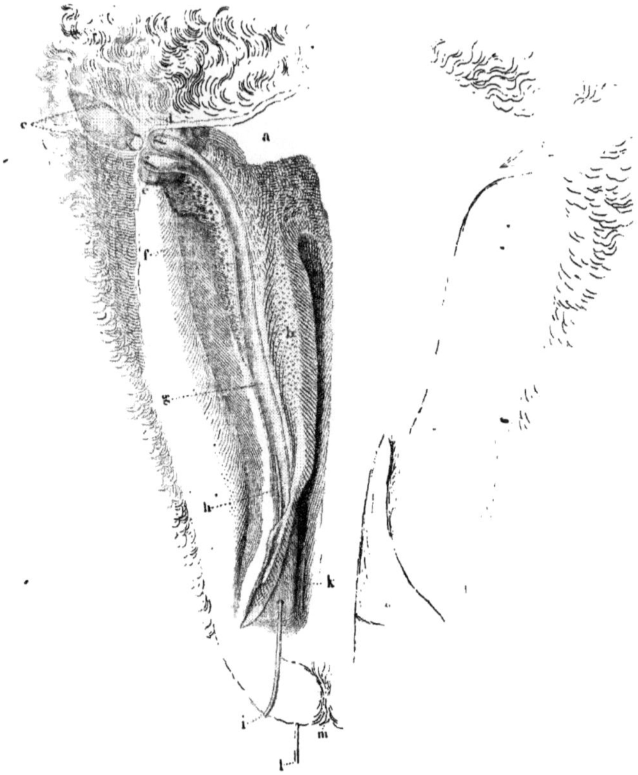

Explanation of Table VIII.

In this Table, the Right Lachrymal Nafal Duct of a Sheep is traced to its Termination in the Nofe; which, when the Face of the Animal is placed horizontally, will be found to be over the Bottom of the Nofe, a very little behind the Upper End of the Ductus Incifivus.

a Reprefents the Os Nafi of the Right Side cut.

b The Os Spongiofum Inferius.

c The Eyelids.

d e Probes paffed through the Puncta Lachrymalia into the Lachrymal Sac.

f g The

f g The Lachrymal Naſal Duct laid open.

h i A Probe paſſed from the Lachrymal Duct into the Cavity of the Noſe.

k l A Probe paſſed through the Canalis Inciſivus.

m The Fiſſure in the Upper Lip.

THE END OF TREATISE SECOND.

OBSERVATIONS

ON THE

ORGAN OF HEARING

IN

MAN

AND OTHER ANIMALS.

BY

ALEXANDER MONRO, M. D.

PROFESSOR OF MEDICINE, ANATOMY, AND SURGERY,

IN THE UNIVERSITY OF EDINBURGH.

EDINBURGH:

PRINTED BY ADAM NEILL AND COMPANY

1797.

A Table of the Contents of Treatise III.

CHAP.

PREFACE.

PREFACE.

SO far back as the year 1756, whilſt I was in Berlin, obſerving, that no Anatomiſt had traced the Diſtribution of the Portio Mollis of the Auditory Nerve within the Cochlea, Veſtible, and Semicircular Canals; or, that the Structure of thoſe principal parts of the Ear on which ultimately Impreſſion is made, and to which all the other pieces of its complex and elegant machinery are ſubſervient, was unknown; I began to inveſtigate the ſubject with accuracy, and ſoon found the means of tracing the progreſs of the Portio Mollis, the minute branches of which I proſecuted upon the Cochlea chiefly.

From that time downwards, I have demonſtrated theſe annually, in my Courſes of Lectures in this Univerſity; and, in 1783, when I publiſhed my Obſervations on the Nervous Syſtem, I gave a Deſcription of theſe Preparations, illuſtrated by Figures, (See Tables XXIX. XXX. & XXXI.); and, before publication, I ſhewed my Preparations to ſeveral excellent judges.

Two years thereafter, in 1785, in a Work I publiſhed on the Structure and Phyſiology of Fiſhes, compared with thoſe of Man and other Animals; I deſcribed the Parts of the Ear in the Whale, in Amphibious Animals, and in Fiſhes; and illuſtrated my Deſcriptions with a Number of Figures. (See Tables VII. XXXIV. XXXV. XXXVI. XXXVII. XXXVIII. & XXXIX.)

Soon thereafter, to-wit in 1787, I received a Letter from the late Dr CAMPER, in which he denies the exiſtence of Semicircular Canals in Whales, and calls in queſtion that of the Meatus Auditorius Externus in the Skate and Squalus Squatina, which I had deſcribed.

I ſhould

I ſhould not have pointed out to the Public what I knew to be erroneous in Dr CAMPER's Letter, if he had not, at the ſame time, written me, that he intended to have his Remarks inſerted into a German Tranſlation of my Book on Fiſhes, which he told me was then about to be publiſhed by Dr SCHNEIDER, " in order to put me right, and to be uſeful to others *."

Still later, in 1787, Dr ANTONIUS SCARPA, Profeſſor of Anatomy and Surgery in Pavia, Ticinum, in a large Work, entitled, " Diſquiſitiones Anatomicæ de Auditu et Olfactu," illuſtrated with many Tables, has repreſented the Deſcription I had given of the Human Ear as inaccurate; and the whole of my Account of the Meatus Auditorius Externus, and of the Communication of it with the Interior Parts of the Ear, and of theſe with each other, in the Cartilaginous Fiſhes, as a mere fiction.

* I obſerve this Tranſlation, by J. G. SCHNEIDER, with Dr CAMPER's Notes, quoted by Dr SOEMMERING as publiſhed, in 1787, at Leipſic; but I have not yet ſeen it.

Although, from the attention I had paid to these subjects, and that I had in my possession the several Preparations from which my Descriptions were taken, and had demonstrated these publicly in my Courses of Lectures, and privately to many good judges of such matters; yet, the reputation which Dr CAMPER and Dr SCARPA have acquired, made it necessary for me, on my own account, and likewise to prevent others from being misled, by their authority, on these highly curious and interesting parts of Anatomy, to resume my researches on these subjects.

The Public will reap the advantage of having these organs more fully described, and of seeing them more elegantly delineated, than in my former Figures, by my assistant Mr FYFE, from recent Preparations, which, at my request, he undertook to make; and which he has, by my direction, executed with great dexterity and accuracy.

All the Preparations from which the Figures I formerly published, or which I now publish, have been taken, are still in my possession. They have all been lately demonstrated to the Members of the Royal Society of this place, and minutely examined by such Members as are best qualified to judge of such subjects, after they were made acquainted with the doubts raiſed by CAMPER and SCARPA, and that their atteſtation as to facts would be requeſted.

I ſhall now proceed to deſcribe the Structure of ſome of the principal Parts of the Ear, in Man and in other Animals; I ſhall then add the atteſtation, as to the accuracy of my Deſcription and Tables, of thoſe Members of the Royal Society, who have examined my Preparations, and Figures taken from them; and I ſhall conclude with a few Obſervations on Profeſſor SCARPA's Work.

TREATISE

TREATISE THIRD:

ON THE EAR.

CHAP. I.

Of the Size, Shape, and relative Situation, of the Cavities of the Ear.

THAT the Size, Shape, and relative Situation, of the Cavities of the Ear, might be more diſtinctly perceived than they can be by cutting the Bones in the common way, I propoſed to my Son, to fill them with Metal, and then to deſtroy the Bone; which he executed very dexterouſly and ſucceſsfully: And in Four Figures of Table I. an exact Repreſentation

Repreſentation is given of his Preparation, from Drawings of it by Mr FYFE; to which, with its Explanation, I ſhall refer the Reader. The Cochlea, in particular, is ſo completely filled as to give an excellent view of its Size and Figure.

In Table II. I have repreſented the appearance of Caverns in different kinds of Quadrupeds, reſembling in office thoſe of our Maſtoid Proceſs. Theſe are, in proportion, conſiderably larger, and their ſides thinner and more elaſtic, than in Man; and there can be no doubt, that the greater Acuteneſs of thoſe Animals in Hearing, is, in part, owing to the Structure of theſe Caverns.

CHAP.

CHAP. II.

Of the Structure of the Human Cochlea.

SECT. I.

IT has been long known, that the Human Cochlea deſcribes two complete *Gyri* or Turns, and a Half Turn; that a central conical oſſeous Pillar, called *Modiolus*, is continued to the Middle of its Second *Gyrus*; that the *Gyri* are divided, by a Partition called *Lamina Spiralis,* into Two Winding Canals, called *Scalæ*; that one *Scala* begins from the Veſtible, and is therefore called *Scala* of the *Veſtible*, and that

 the

the other begins at the *Foramen Rotundum* in the Backpart of the Cavity of the *Tympanum*, and is therefore called the *Scala* of the *Tympanum*; that the *Scalæ* are Wider at the Veſtible and Foramen Rotundum than at the Apex of the Cochlea, or, that they are of a Conical figure; that at the Apex of the Cochlea they communicate with each other, by opening into a Common Tube, called *Infundibulum* or Funnel, one End of which begins at the Termination of the Modiolus, and the other End of it is fixed to the oſſeous Top or Cupola of the Cochlea.

SECT. II.

It is evident, that the Oſſeous Structure of the Human Cochlea muſt be fully explained, before we can deſcribe its Membranes and Courſe of its Nerves; and as ſome material circumſtances have eſcaped the obſervation of Authors, I ſhall give a ſhort Deſcription of this, illuſtrated by Figures.

The Central Pillar of the Cochlea conſiſts of Two Parts, called Modiolus and Infundibulum.

The

The Modiolus is not a ſolid Oſſeous Cone, as has been generally ſuppoſed, but may be conſidered as a Hollow Cone, containing that Branch of the Portio Mollis which is deſtined for the Cochlea; and is everywhere Cribriform, for the Paſſage of the Branches of that Nerve. The Infundibulum is an imperfect Oſſeous Funnel, connected to the Top of the Modiolus. So that the Modiolus and Infundibulum are Two Hollow Conical Bodies, connected together by their ſmall Ends. The Plate which is between them, and in the Centre of both, is Cribriform. Around the Modiolus, the Firſt Gyrus of the Cochlea and Half of the Second Gyrus are deſcribed; the other Half Gyrus incloſes the Root of the Infundibulum; and the Upper Ends of the Gyri, which communicate with each other, are covered or incloſed by the Cupola of the Cochlea.

The Partitions of Bone which ſeparate the Gyri from each other, are not compoſed of One Solid Plate, as Authors have repreſented *, but conſiſt of Two Plates, connected to the Modiolus at ſome diſtance from each other.

 The

* Du Verney.—Cassebohm, T. 5. F. 7, 8, 9, 10.—Scarpa, P. 10. F. 3. 7.

The Offeous Root of the Lamina Spiralis is likewife compofed of Two Plates, connected to the Modiolus or Root of the Infundibulum, at fome diftance from each other.

I have already obferved, that the Modiolus is compofed of a Cribriform Hollow Cone, the Sides of which confift of Two Thin Plates; and the Holes in it are much more Numerous than they have been defcribed to be by Authors, and are not difpofed in the Regular Manner they have reprefented them *.

They are to be feen in every part of the Surface of the Modiolus; but are moft numerous clofe to the Roots of the Offeous Septa which feparate the Gyri from each other; and clofe to the Outer Sides of the Root of the Lamina Spiralis. They are numerous in the Plate between the Modiolus and Infundibulum; and when the Offeous Septa and Lamina Spiralis are cut near the Modiolus, they are feen in the Side of the Modiolus, between the Two Plates which compofe the Septa and Lamina Spiralis.

In

---

* Cassebohm, T. 5. F. 10.

In Table III. the Oſſeous Structure of the Cochlea is accurately repreſented, magnified to Five Diameters; and a full Explanation of it is annexed, to which I ſhall refer the Reader.

SECT. III.

It had been, and ſtill is, generally ſuppoſed, that the Portio Mollis is diſtributed upon the Perioſteum lining the Cochlea and Semicircular Canals: But, the extraordinary Hardneſs and Thickneſs of theſe Bones, the Smallneſs of the Holes by which the Nerves enter, and the great Delicacy and Tenderneſs of the Membranes within the Cochlea,—had prevented Anatomiſts from tracing the Courſe of the Branches of the Portio Mollis within the Os Petroſum, and from perceiving the nature of the Interior Membranes, and the manner in which the Nerves terminate upon theſe.

To

To ſhew the Reader how little was known upon theſe ſubjects, I ſhall quote, at the bottom of the page, the account given of them by the moſt eminent Anatomiſts of the preſent century *.

As

---

* VALSALVA, de Aure Humana, Cap. iii. § 14. "Vidique demum minima "quædam foramina, ... per quæ nerveæ fibrillæ Cochleam ſubeunt. Intra "hanc vero eædem *probabiliter* in membranam expanſæ."

WINSLOW, Exp. An. P. 2. S. x. § 409. 1732. "La Portion Molle du Nerf "Auditif aboutit par ſon tronc à la grande foſſette du Trou Auditif Interne, ou "les filets de ce tronc paſſent par pluſieurs petits troncs de la baſe du Limaçon, "en partie au Perioſte des Canaux demicirculaires, en partie au Perioſte Interne "des demi-canaux du Limaçon." He ſays nothing of their appearance or diſtribution on this *Perioſteum.*

CASSEBOHM, de Aure Humana. 1734. Tr. v. § 227. "Neque in Cochlea "Humana filamentum nerveum unquam obſervavi."

HALLER, El. Phyſ. Lib. xv. § 38. 1763. "Nervum autem aliquem in conſpicua filamenti ſpecie, per Cochlea ſpiras circumduci, (uti pingit VALSALVA), "nunquam vidi. Sed nequidem, manus Anatomicæ, etiam ſumma induſtria, Nervulos ex modiolo per foramina, jam a nobis expoſita, aut in ſcalam cochleæ alterutram, aut in duplicis laminæque ſpiralis membranaceum complementum, efficientis perioſtei intervallum duxerit."

HALLER,

SECT. IV.

As, previous to 1756, when I firſt attempted to trace the Portio Mollis within the Cochlea, I had repeatedly rendered Injected

HALLER, in Pr. Lin. Phyſ. § 493. " Alter ramus, qui Cochleæ ſulcum ſubit, " obſcuram finem habet."

COTUNNIUS, de Aquod. Auris Hum. 1761. § 25. " Continuari tamen hos " nervorum ductus cum canaliculis inter lamellas ſpiralis laminæ deſcriptis (xiv.); " perque hos ad intervallum zonæ cochleæ nervorum ramulos tranſire, etſi pro " ſumma tenuitate rerum *non videam inſpexiſſe*, extra omne tamen dubium aſſeri " poſſe credo. Ultra de hoc nervo me nihil ſcire, ſincerus fateor."

J. FR. MECKEL junior. 1777. § xxiii. p. 40. " Aperto enim cochleæ tubo " a foramine rotundo ad uſque tertium ipſius gyrum, ita ut, ſupra et infra ſep- " tum utraque ſcala perioſteo induta luſtrari potuerit, etiam vitrorum, objecta " multum augentium, miniſterio, nil intueri licuit, niſi albas inter trabeculas Co- " chleæ ſtrias."

MARTIN, de Nervis. 1781. S. 2. p. 82. " Vaſculum aliquod ſanguiferum " pro nervo habitum eſt, vel etiam portiunculæ membranarum filamentorum ſimi- " litudinem retulerunt."

SABATIER. 1781. T. 3. p. 252. " Mes obſervations n'ont pu me donner " des lumieres ſur un choſe auſſi obſcure."

Injected Bones ſoft and tranſparent, and, in doing ſo, had remarked, that, though the Bones were made very Tender, the Membranes connected with them retained a conſiderable degree of Tenacity, it readily occurred to me, that by this means I might be enabled to trace the whole progreſs of the Portio Mollis.

Accordingly my ſucceſs equalled my expectation; and with a great deal of pains I detached the Os Petroſum, and the whole External Oſſeous Shell of the Cochlea from its Interior Membranes; and then took out the Membranes, with the Modiolus and Lamina Spiralis ſuſpended by the Trunk of the Portio Mollis: So that, by proper diſſection, I could trace and ſee diſtinctly, not only the Diviſion of the Portio Mollis into its Larger Branches, but the whole Progreſs and Termination of theſe.

I found, That the Portio Mollis is compoſed of Two Branches nearly equal in ſize; one of which ſupplies the Veſtible and Semicircular Canals, and the other the Cochlea. See Nervous Syſtem, Tab. XXX. Fig. 1, 2, 3, 4, 5.

That each Branch conſiſts of a great Number of Small Cords. See Nervous Syſtem, Tab. XXXI. Fig. 1, 2, 3. A A.

That

That the Small Cords of both Branches paſs through different minute Holes into the Veſtible and Cochlea, or, that the Bottom of the Canal in the Backpart of the Os Petroſum, commonly called Meatus Auditorius Internus, is Cribriform. See Nervous Syſtem, Table XXIX. Fig. 12. X Y Z *cc d e*.

As the Oſſeous Partitions which divide the Cochlea into its Gyri, as well as the Lamina Spiralis which divides the Gyri into Scalæ, are connected to the Circumference of the Modiolus; we might expect to find the Branches of the Portio Mollis conducted, from the Modiolus, to the Membranes lining the Cochlea, by means of theſe Partitions, or between or along the outer-ſides of the Two Oſſeous Plates which compoſe them, as well as between the Two Lamellæ which compoſe the Lamina Spiralis, or along the outer-ſides of theſe; as we would ſuppoſe, that the Two Sides of each Scala ſhould have Nerves diſtributed on them in the ſame manner.

Accordingly, on proſecuting the Branches or Fibres of the Portio Mollis with the utmoſt attention, I find, that they paſs Outwards from the Cavity of the Modiolus, through innumerable minute Holes or Canals, which every where perforate it. Some Fibrils paſs between the Two Plates which form the Septa that ſeparate the Gyri from each other. A ſtill greater number of Fibrils paſſes through Holes between the Two Plates which compoſe the Root of the Lamina Spiralis. But by far the greateſt number of the Nervous Fibrils perforates the Sides of the Modiolus, between the Oſſeous Septa and the Lamina Spiralis. The Fibrils which paſs through the Holes that are neareſt to the Lamina Spiralis, run to the Membrane covering the Lamina Spiralis; whilſt thoſe which are neareſt to the Septa, run, in a contrary direction, to the Membranes covering the Septa. We perceive, therefore, that the part of the Membrane lining each Scala which is the moſt diſtant from the Modiolus, will be ſupplied by the Terminations of theſe Two Sets of Fibrils meeting. The Nervous Fibrils on the Surface of the Lamina Spiralis, ſeem larger, and are more regularly diſpoſed, than thoſe that run on the Surface of the Septa. Two Plates are found in the Outer Oſſeous Part of the Lamina Spiralis, and the Space between them is filled with Nervous Fibres, from which numerous minute Fibrils iſſue between the Outer Edges of the Two Plates. There are likewiſe minute Holes in the Sides of each of the Plates which compoſe the Lamina Spiralis; and there can be no doubt

doubt that the Nerves between the Plates are connected with thofe which run on their External Surface.

The laft Branches or Fibres of the Portio Mollis pafs through the Cribriform Plate, in the Top of the Modiolus, which is common to it and the Infundibulum, to fupply the laft Half-Gyrus and Cupola of the Cochlea. See Nervous Syftem, Table XXXI. Fig. 1, 2, 3. and Table IIII. of this Work.

I next obferved, that the feveral Branches of the Portio Mollis, in their whole courfe along the Lamina Spiralis, formed an elegant and intricate Plexus, by innumerable Joinings and Separations of their component Fibrils. See Nervous Syftem, Tab. XXXI. Fig. 1, 2, 3, 4. and Tab. IIII. Fig. 1, 2, 3.

At the Root or Offeous Part of the Lamina Spiralis, the Nerves are White and Opaque; but at the Flexible and Membranous Parts they are Semipellucid. See Nervous Syftem, Tab. XXXI. Fig. 1, 2, 3, 4. and Tab. III.

This Change of Colour is like to that we obferve the Optic Nerve undergoes on entering the Eyeball to form the

 Retina:

Retina: and, in both, the Change of Colour is not very gradually made, but ſuddenly.

On comparing the Semipellucid Outer-part of the Lamina Spiralis with the Retina of the Eye, I obſerved a remarkable difference; to-wit, that in the Retina the Texture ſeems Pulpy and Uniform, without any ſuch appearance of Fibres and Network as we might expect to obſerve from the name *Retina*, which has been ſo long and univerſally given to it; whereas, in the Ear, Fibres and the Continuation of an intricate Network can be ſeen diſtinctly in the Semipellucid Part of the Lamina Spiralis, and as far as to its Outer Edge. See Nervous Syſtem, Tab. XXXI. Fig. 4. E F G. and Tab. IIII. Fig. 1, 2, 3.

I have, therefore, in my Lectures, long obſerved, that the term *Retina* was improper when applied to the Nerve ſpread out on the Bottom of the Eye, and had been given, not in conſequence of accurate obſervation of the Structure, but from a common favourite theory of Anatomiſts, which ſuppoſes that the Brain and Nerves conſiſt of Fibres. In the Ear, the term may be, with great propriety, applied to deſcribe the Appearance of the Branches of the Portio Mollis in their courſe on the Lamina Spiralis.

At

At the Outer-part of the Lamina Spiralis, the Nervous Fibres and Network become much leſs evident; and, upon the Continuation of theſe Membranes, on the Inner-ſides of the Gyri of the Cochlea, the Nerves ſeem to terminate in a Semipellucid Pulpy Subſtance, very like to the Retina of the Eye.

SECT. V.

I WOULD next obſerve, that the Membrane on which the Branches of the Portio Mollis terminate in the outer tranſparent part of the Lamina Spiralis and on the Inner-ſides of the Gyri of the Cochlea, is not the Perioſteum of the Lamina Spiralis or of the Gyri, as has been univerſally ſuppoſed, but is as different from it as the Pleura is from the Perioſteum of the Ribs. It is thick, ſoft, demipellucid, and but ſlightly connected to the Inner-ſides of the Gyri; and, tracing the Branches of the Portio Mollis, it is evidently formed by them carrying with them their Pia Mater, nearly as the Retina is formed by the Optic Nerve. Beſides, after detaching it from the Inner-ſides of the Gyri, the Bone is ſo far from appearing bare, that we ſee Blood-

veſſels

veſſels running upon its Surface, ſupported by Membrane, which is indeed ſo thin and tender that we cannot eaſily raiſe it by diſſection, but we can ſhew it as diſtinctly as the Perioſteum which lines the Cavity of the Tympanum.

CHAP. III.

Of the Ear in Whales.

SOUND, I formerly obſerved *, is conveyed to the Bottom of the Ears in Whales, by the ſame general Structure as in Man and Quadrupeds.

They are all provided with a Meatus Auditorius Externus, the Orifice into which, in the Cete Delphinus, is extremely ſmall; and it appears to me probable, that they poſſeſs the power of ſhutting it, and excluding the water, when they plunge to a conſiderable depth. In the Cete Balæna, (1. of LINNEUS), the largeſt of the Whale kind, there is within the

* In my Book on Fiſhes.

the Meatus Auditorius a Hard Body, upwards of an Inch in Length, ſhaped like an Egg, and attached by its ſmall end to one ſide of the Meatus; which undoubtedly ſerves as a Valve, to prevent the Water, when the Whale dives deep, from over-diſtending and rupturing the Membrane of the Drum †.

Their Membrana Tympani is tied by a Chain of Bones to the Bottom of the Tympanum; but in this Chain the Os *Orbiculare* is wanting, at leaſt it is ſo in the Phyſeter; and the Malleus is more fixed in its place than in Man.

I found, that they have likewiſe an Euſtachian Tube, or Internal Meatus Auditorius; and that Cells, much larger in proportion than thoſe of our Maſtoid Proceſs, communicate with the Cavity of their Tympanum. See Tab. V. Fig. 5. and Tab. XXXV. Fig. 5, 6. on Fiſhes.

Their Cochlea and Semicircular Canals, I obſerved, were analogous to ours.

When

† See, in Table VI. *, a Figure of this, of its Natural Size, taken from a Preparation I received lately from Mr CLAPERTON.

When I firſt publiſhed on the ſubject, I thought it unneceſſary to trace their Semicircular Canals with accuracy. But finding, by Dr CAMPER's Letter, that he, after having diſſected various Species of the Whale, perſiſted in denying their exiſtence, I have reſumed the ſubject with greater attention: And, after finding that I had been under no miſtake in deſcribing Semicircular Canals, I aſked Mr FYFE to beſtow ſome pains in tracing their whole Extent, firſt in the Delphinus Phocæna, and afterwards in the Delphinus Delphis, and in the Cete Phyſeter Macrocephalus or Spermaceti Whale, which laſt Dr CAMPER had diſſected; and to draw accurate Figures of them; to which, and their Explanation, I refer the Reader. See Tab. V. and Tab. VI.

On viewing theſe Figures, the Reader will obſerve, that the Cochlea in the Cete Phyſeter is much larger than in Man, but that the Semicircular Canals are ſmaller: And, ſo far as I have examined the Ear, I have found, that the Semicircular Canals in Man, bear a larger proportion to the Cochlea, than they do in the Quadruped or Whale.

CHAP. IV.

Of the Ear in Cartilaginous Fishes.

BEFORE I published my Work on Fishes, I had examined this subject with great attention; and have the satisfaction to find, on repeating my experiments, that my observations were correct in every respect: So that the descriptions I am about to give, contain a repetition of what I formerly published, but illustrated with more elegant Figures drawn by Mr FYFE.

I ſhall confine my deſcriptions chiefly, and almoſt entirely, to the Skate Fiſh *.

In the upper and back part of the Head of a Skate, and in a large Fiſh weighing 150 pounds, at the diſtance nearly of One Inch from the Articulation of the Head with the Firſt Vertebra of the Neck or Atlas, Two Orifices, capable of admitting ſmall-ſized ſtocking-wires, at the diſtance of about an Inch and Quarter from each other, ſurrounded with a firm membranous Ring, may be obſerved. See Tab. VII. Fig. 1, 2, 3. Letters *a a a a*. Theſe are the Beginnings of the Meatus Auditorii Externi.

If the Finger be applied a little farther forwards and inwards than one of theſe Orifices, and Preſſure made with it, a White Viſcid Matter will generally be ſqueezed out at the Orifice.

If

* See Tab. VII. in the Firſt Figure of which the parts are repreſented as they appear on diſſection. In Figures Second and Third, they are repreſented as they appeared, in a Fiſh weighing 150 pounds, after being ſtretched with melted wax injected into them.

If a Small Probe be introduced at the Orifice, and a Cut made upon the Point of the Probe, we discover a Winding Canal, nearly two lines, or the sixth part of an inch, in Diameter, which describes more than three-fourths of a Circle. See the same Figures, Letters *b b b b*. This Winding Canal may be compared to the Concha of our External Ear.

From the Concha, a Straight Passage, capable of admitting a small stocking-wire, leads outwards and downwards, (See in the same Figures the Letters *c c c*), to terminate in a Large Sac *d d d d*; which we may compare to the Vestible in the Human Body; and which, in the Skate, contains a very viscid pellucid Humour, like the glaire of an egg, and likewise a soft cretaceous Substance.

On the anterior part of the Large Sac, there is a much Smaller Sac *e e e e*, containing similar Matter, and communicating freely with the Large Sac at the Letters *f f f f*; and at the posterior part, there is a third very Small Bag, likewise containing cretaceous Matter, projecting from and communicating with the Large Bag.

We next find Three Semicircular, or rather Circular, Membranous Canals. In each of them, there is a Bulb or dilated.

ted part. All of them are incloſed within Cartilaginous Canals, lined with Perichondrium, which are conſiderably larger than the Membranous Canals. The Membranous Canals are filled with viſcid pellucid Humour, like to that which is within the Veſtible; and a Fluid reſembling this, is lodged between the Perichondrium and the Membranous Canals; and theſe are tied to each other by Cellular Threads, on which Arteries, correſponding Veins, Lympha-tics, and very minute Nerves, are diſperſed. See Table XXXVII. Fig. 4. of my Work on Fiſhes.

One of theſe Canals is Anterior, See Tab. VII. Fig. 1, 2, 3. Letters *h i k l o*; and the part *k* is almoſt over the part *o*, or this Canal may be called Anterior Perpendicular: At *l* its Bulb is found. The Second or Middle Canal *m n*, is placed almoſt horizontally; and its Bulb is ſeen at *n*.

The Anterior and Horizontal Canals join together, and the wide Canal *i h o* is common to them. This Canal, common to the Anterior and Horizontal Canals, commu-nicates with the Small Sac *e*, by means of the Membranous Tube *g*.

The

The Third Circular Canal is Poſterior, and one half of it is over the other; ſo that it may be called Poſterior Perpendicular Canal. See *q r ſ*. Its Bulb is at *ſ*. This Canal communicates with the Large Sac or Veſtible, by means of the Duct *p*; but has no direct communication with either of the other two Circular Canals.

Upon the whole, then,—The Meatus Auditorius Externus leads to the Cavity of the Veſtible. From this there is a Paſſage into a Smaller Sac, and, at the ſame place, a Duct leads into the Membranous Canal which is common to the Anterior and Horizontal Canals. From the Poſterior Part of the Veſtible, a Canal makes a Communication between the Veſtible and the Poſterior Canal. But the Anterior and the Horizontal Canal have no direct Communication with the Poſterior Canal.

It appears, then, that from the Meatus Auditorius there is a Paſſage into the Large Sac or Veſtible; and that from the Forepart of the Veſtible, there is a Paſſage into the Small Sac, and, at the ſame place, into the Canal which is common to the Anterior and Horizontal Canals; and that, from the Backpart of the Large Sac or Veſtible, there is a Paſſage

Paſſage into the Poſterior Canal; and, hence, that all parts of the Veſtible and Circular Canals may be directly affected, in the living animal, or, after death, may be injected, through the Meatus Auditorius Externus.

CHAP.

CHAP. V.

Summary of the Chief Circumſtances above deſcribed.

AS ſeveral of the principal Facts I have deſcribed, have, moſt unaccountably, been called in queſtion, by Dr CAMPER and Profeſſor SCARPA, I find myſelf under the diſagreeable neceſſity of enumerating, in a ſummary way, the Chief Points, reſpecting the Organ of Hearing in Man and other Animals, in which, I apprehend, I have added to the former ſtock of knowledge; and of then ſubjoining the Atteſtation of the Royal Society of Edinburgh concerning them.

A. In the Human Body, I have ſhewed, That the Nerves of the Veſtible and Semicircular Canals, as well as thoſe of the Cochlea, paſs through numerous Small Holes or Cribriform Plates of the Os Petroſum *.

B. That all the Branches of the Portio Mollis which ſupply the Cochlea, paſs through innumerable Small Holes of a Thin Conical Cribriform Plate which forms the Modiolus †.

C. That minute Nerves paſs through the Axis of the Modiolus, to perforate that part of the Cribriform Plate which is common to it and to the Infundibulum, to ſupply the Infundibulum and that part of the Cochlea which it includes ‡.

D. That

---

* See Nervous Syſtem, Tab. XXIX.

† See Nervous Syſtem, Tab. XXIX.

‡ See Nervous Syſtem, Tab. XXXI.

D. That Branches of the Portio Mollis paſs along and between the Lamellæ of the Oſſeous Septa which divide the Cochlea into its Gyri *; or, that all of them are not conducted by the Lamina Spiralis, as SCARPA has deſcribed and delineated †.

E. That the Nerves, in their whole courſe, particularly along the Lamina Spiralis, join and again are ſeparated, ſo as to form a moſt elegant Plexus; in which new Combinations of the Nerves are formed ‡.

F. That the Nerves terminate on the Inner-ſides of the Oſſeous Gyri, in a demipellucid ſoft pulpy Membrane, reſembling the Retina of the Eye ‖.

* See Nervous Syſtem, Tab. XXXI. and, of this Treatiſe, Tab. IIII.

† SCARPA, P. 55. and Tab. VIII.

‡ See Nervous Syſtem, Tab, XXXI.

‖ See Nervous Syſtem, Tab. XXXI. and, of this Treatiſe, Tab. III.

G. That this ſoft pulpy Membrane is not the Perioſteum of the Cochlea; but as different from it, as the Pleura is from the Perioſteum of the Ribs.

H. In Whales, I have found an Euſtachian Tube, which had not been deſcribed by Authors: I have ſhewn, that Semicircular Canals are not wanting, as was affirmed by Dr CAMPER; and, in the Porpoiſe, I obſerved, that the Membranous Subſtance, within the Gyri of the Cochlea, on which the Portio Mollis is diſtributed, might be ſeparated from the Perioſteum of the Cochlea ſtill more eaſily than in Man *.

I. In the Tortoiſe, as an example of the Amphibia, I have deſcribed the Euſtachian Tubes, and the Connexion of the ſeveral parts of the Ear, more accurately than had been done by former Authors †: And it may be worth while to add, that the Toad, as well as the Frog, is provided with an Euſtachian Tube, as this is denied by GEOFFROY ‡.

K. In

* See Book on Fiſhes, Tab. XXXV. and, of this Treatiſe, Tab. V.

† See Book on Fiſhes, Tab. XXXVI.

‡ GEOFFROY ſur l'Organe de l'Ouïe, 1778, p. 65,—71.

K. In ſome of the Piſces of LINNÆUS, I have not only deſcribed and painted the Connexion of the Semicircular Canals, and of Sacs which may be compared to our Veſtible; but I have traced, with accuracy, the Courſe and Termination of their Nerves *.

L. In the Skate and Angel Fiſh, I have diſcovered the Orifices of the Meatus Auditorii; ſhewn the Winding of their Conchæ Aurium; the Terminations of their Meatus Auditorii in the Veſtibles; the Communications of their Semicircular Canals with each other and with the Veſtibles; and Diſtribution of their Auditory Nerves, and of the Circulating and Lymphatic Veſſels of their Ears †.

M. Particularly, I proved, that the Semicircular Canals in Fiſhes were much ſmaller than the Oſſeous or Cartilaginous Tubes which incloſed them; and that, ſo far from their being compoſed of the Perioſteum or Perichondrium of theſe Canals, there was a conſiderable Space between

* See Book on Fiſhes, Tab. XXXIX.

† See Book on Fiſhes, Tab. VII. XXXVII. XXXVIII. and, of this Treatiſe, Tab. VI. VII.

between them, and the Periosteum or Perichondrium, filled with Fluid, contained in a Cellular Substance, on which minute Nerves, with numerous Circulating and Absorbing Vessels, were dispersed, and conducted to the Perichondrium and Periosteum *. I observed farther, That in certain Fishes, of the genus Gadus, Spheroidal Bodies, which I had discovered, making in them part of the Nervous System, were dispersed in the Cellular Substance, between the Semicircular Canals and the Periosteum of the Tubes which contain them †.

* See Book on Fishes, Tab. XXXVII. XXXVIII. XXXIX.

† See Book on Fishes, Tab. XXXIX.

CHAP. VI.

Atteſtation as to the Facts above deſcribed.

HAVING fully deſcribed, and illuſtrated by Tables, the Chief Parts of the Ear in the different Claſſes of Animals; and having enumerated the particular Circumſtances I have diſcovered which were unknown to former Writers; I ſhall now add the Atteſtation of the Royal Society of Edinburgh reſpecting ſuch facts as have been called in queſtion by Dr CAMPER and Profeſſor SCARPA.

At

At their Meeting, in May 1794, I presented to the Society the following Letter:

" Gentlemen,

" AS one purpose of your Society is to ascertain such " Facts as are described by your Members or Correspondents, " I take this liberty to request of you to appoint a Commit- " tee, consisting of those Members whom you may suppose to " be the most competent Judges of Anatomical Matters, to " examine certain Subjects of which I propose to give, soon, " some account to the Society, illustrated with Figures.

" I am,

" Gentlemen,

" Your most obedient Servant,

Edinburgh, May 2. 1794.

" Alex^r. Monro.

" To the President and Other Members of the Royal " Society."

They accordingly appointed a large Committee of their number, with a general invitation to any others of their Members who might choose to be present.

In consequence of this, the following Gentlemen met, on the 9th of July 1794, in the Anatomical Theatre, at Mid-day, that they might have the advantage of examining my Dissections and Preparations with a clear light:

Mr John Robison, Professor of Natural Philosophy.
Mr Dugald Stewart, Professor of Moral Philosophy.
Mr Playfair, Professor of Mathematics.
Dr Black,
Dr Francis Home,
Dr Rutherford, } Professors of Medicine.
Dr Gregory,
Dr Duncan,
Dr Rotheram, Physician.
Dr Wright, Physician.
Dr Charles Stuart, Physician.
Dr Thomas Spens, Physician.
Mr James Russel, Surgeon.

Along with each of the Figures which I now publifh, I demonftrated the Preparation from which it was delineated: And it is to be obferved, that, in the Cartilaginous Fifhes, I had injected, from the Orifice of their Meatus Auditorius Externus, not only Air and Quickfilver, but melted coloured Wax, into their Veftible and Semicircular Canals; and that I have about twenty fuch Preparations in my poffeffion.

The Committee, after having attentively examined thefe, hereby declare, That the Tables and Preparations correfpond exactly; and that they faw diftinctly, in the Preparations, all that is reprefented in the Tables.

1795. May 14.

On the 14th day of May 1795, I made the following Demonftration to my Colleagues, Dr Home, Dr Gregory, Dr Rutherford, and Dr Duncan.

In Two Large Skates, one the Raia Lævis, the other the Raia Afpera or Thornback, I pointed out, with a Probe, the Orifices of the Meatus Auditorii Externi.

I then

I then preſſed with my finger on the Fore and Inner Sides of theſe Orifices, and ſhewed them, that a white viſcid Matter was diſcharged from them.

A Section was next made on the Right Side of both Fiſhes, and the Veſtible and Semicircular Canals of the Ear were laid in view, without opening their Cavities.

A Small Iron Tube, fixed to a Large Glaſs Tube, was then introduced into the Orifice of the External Meatus Auditorius, and Quickſilver was poured into the Glaſs Tube. The Quickſilver entered readily, and filled the Concha, and ſtretched the Skin over it; ſo that its Shape, Size, and Winding, could be eaſily diſtinguiſhed. From the Concha, the Quickſilver paſſed readily into, and diſtended, the Great Sac, which contains the Cretaceous Matter.—The Paſſage of the Quickſilver from the Meatus Externus Auditorius into the Sac or Veſtible, was ſeen diſtinctly; becauſe the Meatus terminates in that part of the Veſtible which contains the clear viſcid Matter, which is lodged between the upper and outer or poſterior part of the Sac of the Veſtible and the Cretaceous Matter.

They again examined the ſeveral Preparations in which the Concha, Meatus Auditorius, Veſtible and Semicircular Canals, are filled with Wax of different colours in order to ſhew the Communication of theſe Parts, and they compared the Tables with the Preparations.

CHAP.

CHAP. VII.

Remarks on Profeſſor SCARPA's Book on the Ear.

BEFORE concluding, I find myſelf under the diſagreeable neceſſity of pointing out the Injuſtice of certain Criticiſms of Profeſſor SCARPA, and of enumerating the many unaccountable Overſights and Errors he has committed; and I ſhall quote the expreſſions he has thought himſelf at liberty to employ.

SECT.

SECT. I.

In his Preface, p. 3. l. 25. he has aſſerted: "Nam "quidquid nuperrimè Monrous docuit de Acuſtici Nervi "Diſtributione per Laminam Cochleæ Spiralem, nihil aliud "eſt præter mirificæ fabricæ ſpecimen; nec qua ratione "Auditorius Nervus ad Utrumque Scalarum Cochleæ Gyrum "pertingat, nec quo abeat Nervus ille qui per Centrum et "Axin Modioli deſcendit, Vir alioquin cl., nobis patefe- "cit."

The Reader, however, will obſerve, that I have not only every year, ſince 1756, ſhewed, in my Anatomical Courſes, the Preparation from which the Figure I publiſhed was delineated; but that it was particularly examined, before I publiſhed, by the following Gentlemen: Dr Smith, Reader of Anatomy in Oxford; Dr Soemmering, Dr Meckel junior, Mr Luther, Dr Black, Dr Hutton, Dr Rutherford: (See my Book on the Nervous Syſtem, p. 45.): And that I ſtill preſerve the Preparation; and, on examining it again, after reading the above aſſertion, I find nothing materially

terially wrong in the Figure.——But, what is more directly in point, so inconsistent is Dr Scarpa, that, in the 55th page of his Work, where he describes the Pencils of Nerves passing from the Modiolus along the Lamina Spiralis, he quotes my Book in the following words: "Horum Penicillorum "specimen vide apud Monroum, Nerv. Syst." And if the Reader will take the trouble of comparing the Figures I published, (See Nervous System, Tab. XXXI. Fig. 1, 2, 3, 4.), with Professor Scarpa's Figures, (Nat. Disq. Tab. VII. Fig. 1, 2.), he will find, that they correspond so much, in every general and material respect, that His Figure seems little more than the Transcript of mine. They differ chiefly in the way in which the Nerves are presented to view. In my Preparation, I took off, with great pains, the whole Outer Osseous Shell of the Cochlea, and then lifted out the Modiolus and Lamina Spiralis, suspended by the Portio Mollis; so that the whole Distribution of the Nerve on the Lamina Spiralis is seen: Whereas Professor Scarpa has cut open one side only of the Cochlea.

I will farther venture to assert, that although Professor Scarpa's Figures are more shewy and elegant than my first Figures.

Figures were, yet mine give a more diſtinct and accurate Repreſentation of Nature.

He next alleges, That I had not ſhewn how the Nerves go to the Gyri of the Cochlea, as if he had ſhewn this better than I had done. But let the Reader compare our Figures; he will find, that Profeſſor SCARPA does not paint the Nerves ſo far as I had done in my Book on the Nervous Syſtem. I painted them as far as diſtinct Branches could be ſeen with a Microſcope which magnified the object to thirty diameters. My deſcriptions, when I publiſhed on the Nervous Syſtem, were indeed very conciſe; becauſe I had the intention of proſecuting the ſubject ſtill more fully than I had then done.

In the next place, it is to be remarked, that One-half of the Nerves the Scalæ of the Cochlea receive, has eſcaped the obſervation of Profeſſor SCARPA *, to wit, All thoſe which run along the Oſſeous Septa to ſupply the Outer-part of each Scala, or that Part of each Scala which is moſt diſtant from the Lamina Spiralis.

But

* See SCARPA, Cap. III. De Nervo Auditorio, § viii.—xii. p. 54, 55, 56.

But I muſt farther obſerve, that Profeſſor SCARPA, who deſcribes the Portio Mollis as terminating in the Perioſteum of the Cochlea, has neither attended properly to the Analogy of the Optic Nerves, nor to the Structure of the Membranes within the Cochlea; for, from the deſcription and reaſons I have given, it is evident, that the Perioſteum, and the Pulpy Membrane in which the Portio Mollis of the Cochlea terminates, are Diſtinct Membranes, the former having the Common Structure, and the latter reſembling the Retina of the Eye.

SECT. II.

In my Book on Fiſhes, p. 49. I obſerved, That in each of the Membranous Semicircular Canals, both in the Oſſeous and in the Cartilaginous Fiſhes, there is a Dilatation or Pouch: and, That the Membranous Canals are ſo much ſmaller, than the Canals of Cartilage or Bone which contain them; that, between them and the Cartilage or Bone, there is a viſcid watery Liquor, contained in a Cellular Subſtance, on the Threads of which, Circulating and Abſorbent Veſſels, and Nerves, are diſperſed. (*b.*) See Tab. XXXVII.

 I likewiſe,

I likewiſe, after deſcribing the Size and Courſe of the Nerves, obſerved, in treating of the Cartilaginous Fiſhes, That "the Nerves, after reaching the Sacs and Canals, and "running a little way upon their Membranes, loſe their "White Colour, become Pellucid, and diſappear." In Tab. XXXVII. theſe Nerves are delineated from very large Fiſhes. And, ſpeaking of the Oſſeous Fiſhes, p. 51. I obſerved, That "very large Nerves are fixed to the *Bulbous* "Parts of the Semicircular Canals, and, ſpreading out on "theſe Canals, they become ſuddenly Pellucid." See Tab. XXXIX.

Still, however, other purſuits diverted me from the intention I had long had, of tracing the whole Diſtribution of the Portio Mollis in the Human Ear.

In 1789, that is, four years after my Book on Fiſhes appeared, Profeſſor SCARPA publiſhed his Deſcription of the Membranes and Nerves of the Human Semicircular Canals: And, although it is evident, as he does not appear to have known any thing of the matter when he publiſhed his "Obſervationes de Feneſtra Rotunda et Tympano Secundario" in 1772, and as he had then read my Works on the Nervous Syſtem and on Fiſhes, that he was led by the firſt of theſe

theſe to examine the Nerves of the Cochlea, and, on the ſuppoſition of analogy, to examine the Veſtible and Semicircular Canals in Man; yet, inſtead of acknowledging this, he tries to inſinuate, that I had not traced the Nerves of the Semicircular Canals in Fiſhes to their proper places, in order to give the appearance of originality to his own deſcriptions. Yet, after joining me with Mr JOHN HUNTER as the author of an aſſertion which Mr HUNTER alone made, —where he ſays, (in a note, p. 15.) " J. HUNTERUS et MONROUS aſſeruerunt Canales Piſcium Semicirculares, Nervos " intus non ſuſcipere;" adding, " Qua ſuper re vereor quàm " maximè Viros cl. examinaſſe tantummodo Cylindros, non " quidem, *Ampullas* ſimul Canalium Semicircularium in Piſci- " bus,"—he, in the ſame note, refutes the truth of his allegation, by ſubjoining the following quotation from my Book: " Et MONROUS, loc. cit. " After reaching the *Sacs* and Ca- " nals, and running a little way upon their Membranes, " they loſe their white colour, become pellucid, and diſap- " pear." And with this deſcription of mine, that of Profeſſor SCARPA exactly coincides: (See his Work, p. 34. § vi. l. 7.): " Neque enim in Homine, proſpero magis ſuc- " ceſſu quàm in Piſcibus, Reptilibus, et Avibus, quantacun- " que adhibita diligentia, datum nobis fuit eam Pulpam, ul-

" tra Ampullaram fines, per continuos semicirculares Ductus " membranaceos, propagatam videre."

In Tab. VIII. Fig. 1, 2, 3. the Reader will find a more exact Representation of the Division of the Acoustic Nerve upon the Ampulla than Professor SCARPA could have given, as it can be seen in very Large Fishes only; which the rude and inaccurate Figure he has published, shews he had not examined.

SECT. III.

PROFESSOR SCARPA, dissatisfied with the account I had given of the Structure of the Ear in the Cartilaginous Fishes, undertakes one more accurate, and has expressed himself in the following terms. His criticisms are strangely disjoined, and unnecessarily repeated; but I shall endeavour to arrange them so as to render them as intelligible as possible.

Præf.

Præf. p. 2. " Has ob caufas Organi Auditus Cartilagi-
" neorum Pifcium pleniorem, quàm adhuc factum eft, de-
" fcriptionem tradere fufcepimus."

Præf. p. 1. " MONROUS Externum hoc Auditus Oftium
" (Rajæ) defcripferit, fufiùs atque delineaverit. . . . .
" MONROUM vehementer fuper hac re hallucinatum fuiffe.
" . . . . . . Etenim nullum prorfus adeft *Oftium* Auditus *extus*
" *Adapertum* in Cartilagineis Pifcibus, ejusque loco, fub Af-
" pero horum Animantium Tegumento, *Feneftra Ovalis* repe-
" riunda eft, *Membranaceo Operculo*, a nemine adhuc memo-
" rato, obducta."

P. 8. § iii. " In Cartilagineis Pifcibus nullum prorfus adeft
" Oftium Auditus extus Adapertum, ejusque prænunciati *Oftii*
" loco, fub communibus tegumentis, *Feneftram Ovalem, Operculo*
" Membranaceo claufam, oftendimus," &c.

P. 9. § v. " Igitur in Summitate Capitis Rajæ ponè Oc-
" ciput, qua nempè cum Prima Colli Vertebra Colli nectitur,
" ablato Spinofo Tegumento, ... Sinuofitas occurrit, in
" qua Membranulæ Duæ, ovalis figuræ Tympani ad modum
" tenfæ, confpiciendæ funt. . . . .

P. 9.

P. 9. § v. in a note at the foot of the page. " MONROUS, " in Opere cui titulus " Phyfiology of Fifhes," Sect. III. " Tab. VII. Fig. 1, 2. docet in Raja, propè Juncturam Capi- " tis cum Spina, adeffe Foramina duo exigua, quæ ad Aures " ducunt. Qua in re vehementer fibi hallucinatus eft; Oftia " nimirùm Ductuum Mucoforum, ut manifeftum eft, pro Au- " ris Meatibus accipiens. Etenim omninò nullum eft in " Cartilagineis Pifcibus Oftium Auditus extus Adapertum, " Membranaque Feneftræ Ovalis fub Communi Tegumento " recondita jacet et cooperta."

P. 9. § vi. Note *(d.)*. " Minimè tamen ducit intra Ca- " vitates Sacculorum Veftibuli, quemadmodum MONROO vi- " fum eft; cujus doctrina, fi vera effet, fimulque adeffent " Oftia Auditus Externa, neceffariò confequeretur liberum ef- " fe in Cartilagineis Pifcibus Aëri et Aquæ Acceffum ad fe- " dem Organi Auditus immediati, ipfamque Pulpam Nervi " Auditorii; quod et abfurdum eft, et a rei veritate quàm " maximè alienum!"

Præf. p. 2. " Præterea, MONROUS nefcio quam Organi " Auditus Cartilagineorum Pifcium hiftoriam confcripfit, ut, " nifi vehementer fallimur, ex ipfius fententia deducere uni-

" cuique

" cuique liceat in Piſcibus Cartilagineis *Meatum* Auditus *Ex-*
" *ternum* ducere intra Sacculos Capillorum, atque ab his ad
" Canales Semicirculares, Nervumque Auditorium; proin,
" Aquis admixtisque heterogeneis particulis nullatenùs in
" Cartilagineis Piſcibus impeditam viam eſſe ab *Externo* (ut
" ait) Auris *Meatu*, ad immediatam Auditus ſedem; quæ res
" profectò a veritate et perſpecta Naturæ providentia quàm
" longiſſimè diſtat!"

P. 12. § xv. " Interim præſtabit monere, Canales Semi-
" circulares Membranoſos, quamvis pluribus in ſedibus La-
" pillorum Sacculis alligati ſunt, nullibi tamen cum iiſdem
" Sacculis communicare; quod *iteratis* periculis, modò
" Aërem, ſervata naturali ſede, per Canales Semicirculares
" Membranoſos inſufflando, modò Hydrargyrum injiciendo,
" cognovimus." —— Note *(e.)*. " Minimè ignoramus Mon-
" roum in Raja deſcripſiſſe ac delineaſſe."

From the above quotations, then, it appears, that Profeſſor Scarpa, even after having read and ſtudied the Deſcription and Figures I had given of the Structure of the Ear in the Skate, illuſtrated by a number of Tables, had not been able to diſcover the External Mouth, or Ostium, of the Meatus Auditorius;

Auditorius; the Concha Auris; the Continuation of the Meatus Auditorius; the Termination of it in the Veſtible, or Large Sac, containing viſcid and cretaceous matter; the Communication of the Large Sac, or Veſtible, with the Smaller Sac, nor the Communication of the Semicircular Canals with theſe Sacs or Veſtibles. Yet, in my experiments, not only Air and Quickſilver readily paſſed in all directions; but, in a great number of Preparations in my poſſeſſion, all the Paſſages and Communications I deſcribed in my former Work, are filled with melted and coloured Wax, and were diſtinctly ſeen by every Member of the Committee of the Royal Society of this place, and by many Students who have examined them.

One thing only, which might be apt to ſtagger ſuch as have not had the opportunity of ſeeing my Preparations, remains to be explained; I mean what relates to a *Feneſtra Ovalis*, which is mentioned by Profeſſor Scarpa, "*Membra-* "*naceo Operculo* obducta, a nemine adhuc memorata."

If the Reader will compare my Book on Fiſhes, Tab. XXXVII. Fig. 2. with Profeſſor Scarpa's, Tab. I. Fig. 1. *e e*, he may obſerve this Feneſtra delineated by me, and a large

large pin ſtuck through it, with the following explanation; page 115. l. 22. " Behind the Concha, there is a Large Soft " Part, which is ſhewn by a pin ſtuck through it." I did not call it Feneſtra Ovalis; becauſe, as I had diſcovered a Meatus Auditorius Externus leading into the Cavity of the Veſtible, I was certain it had no analogy to our Feneſtra Ovalis: And Dr SCARPA, though ignorant of the exiſtence of the Meatus Externus, might have perceived that it did not reſemble the Structure of the Tortoiſe, to which he compares it, (in p. 16. § xxvii. l. 23.); for, as he immediately afterwards obſerves, (l. 27.) " In Cartilagineis Piſcibus mox " retrò Membranam Feneſtræ Ovalis omiſit Natura Oſſiculum, " quòd in Reptilibus pleriſque altera extremitate Tympano " nexum eſt, altera, ſtapedis ad modum, Feneſtram Ovalem " obſtruit."

In Table VI. Fig. 2, 3, 4. T. I have given a ſtill more exact Repreſentation of this Soft Part.

I then ſuppoſed, and ſtill do ſuppoſe, that Nature has formed one part of the Caſe which contains the Veſtible and Semicircular Canals, Soft and Flexible, in order that, by its yielding, the Parts within might be ſuſceptible of Tremulous

 Motion

Motion when Sound acts upon them through the Meatus Auditorius Externus.

After eſtabliſhing the fact, that the Skate and Squalus Squatina are provided with a Meatus Auditorius Externus, it muſt ſeem very ſuperfluous to the Reader to take any notice of what Profeſſor SCARPA has ſtated about the danger of Water and Heterogeneous Matter getting into the Veſtible and Semicircular Canals, injuring the Auditory Nerve, &c.: Yet, I cannot help obſerving, that Profeſſor SCARPA ſeems to have forgotten, not only that the Orifice of the Meatus is like that of the Whale; but likewiſe, that, from the Obliquity of the Meatus or Concha under the Skin, there is no more danger of Air, Water, Sand, &c. getting into the Ear, than there is, that the Drink, the Chyle, or the Urine, ſhall get into the Salivary or Biliary Ducts or Ureters; and likewiſe, that theſe Parts are quite full of Viſcid Matter incloſed in Membranes, incaſed in Thick Cartilages, which therefore will reſiſt the entrance of external Fluids or Solids.

Were

Were it worth while, I might obſerve farther to him, That I have, in the very ſame Animal, diſcovered and deſcribed two much larger Paſſages, with open Orifices, by which the Cavity of the Abdomen communicates with the Water of the Ocean; and, again, within the Animal, Tubes by which the Cavity of the Pericardium communicates with the Cavity of the Abdomen; yet the Interior Parts ſuffer no Injury *.

---

* See my Book on Fiſhes, Tab. XVIII. 10, 11. 29, 30.

TAB. I.

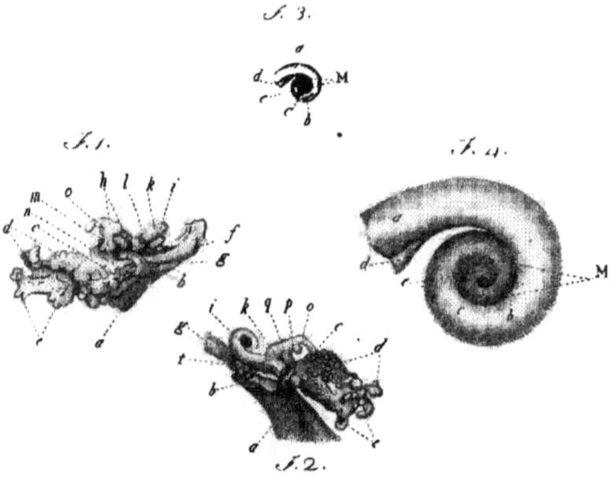

EXPLANATION

OF THE

TABLES.

Explanation of Table I.

THE Figures in this Table give an accurate Repreſentation of Metal, with which the Cavities of the Human Ear, on the Right Side of the Body, had been filled.

FIG. 1, 2.

Fig. 1. repreſents the Forepart of the Metal, and Fig. 2. the Backpart of it.

a Repreſents

a Represents the Metal which filled the Osseous Part of the Meatus Auditorius Externus.

b The Ring where the Membrana Tympani was connected.

T The Cavity of the Tympanum filled.

c The Root of the Cells of the Mastoid Process where they communicate with the Cavity of the Tympanum.

d e The Metal which filled the Cells of the Mastoid Process.

f (Fig. 1.) The Canal filled which contained the Tensor Membrana Tympani.

g The Outer Osseous End of the Eustachian Tube filled.

h The Vestible filled.

i The

i The Cochlea completely filled.

k The Root of the Scala Tympani of the Cochlea.

l The Root of its Scala Veſtibuli.

m (Fig. 1.) The Forepart of the Beginning of the Anterior Perpendicular Semicircular Canal filled.

n (Fig. 1.) The Forepart of the Beginning of the Horizontal Semicircular Canal filled.

o The Canal common to the Two Perpendicular Semicircular Canals filled.

p q (Fig. 2.) At the Places to which the dotted lines, drawn from *p* and *q*, lead, the other Ends of the Poſterior, Perpendicular, and Horizontal, Semicircular Canals, are repreſented, filled with the Metal.

FIG.

FIG. 3, 4.

Fig. 3. ſhews the Metal with which the Cochlea had been filled, as it appears when we look into the Conical Cavity M, which the Modiolus had occupied, and which was not filled with the Metal.

Fig. 4. gives the ſame view of the Preparation magnified to Four Diameters.

a b c The Scala of the Tympanum filled.

d e Part of the Scala of the Veſtibulum ſeen in this view. The reſt of it, is hid by the Scala of the Tympanum.

Explanation

TAB. II.

Fig. 1.

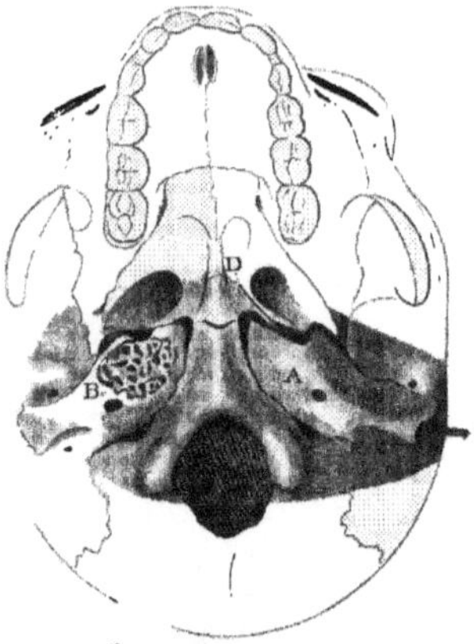

F. 2.

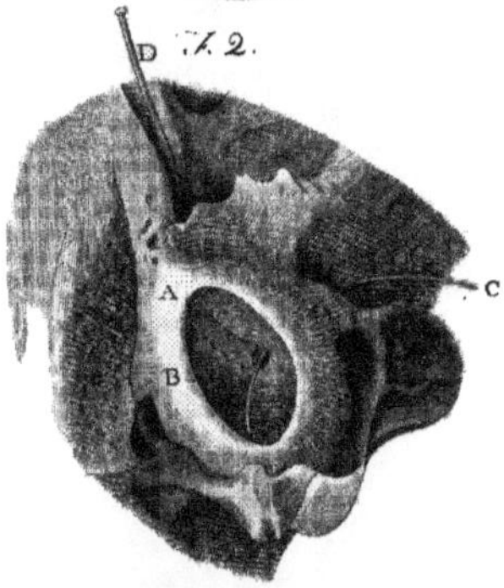

F. 3

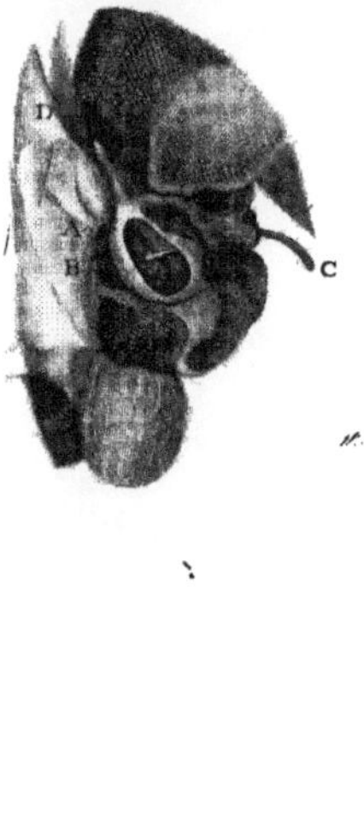

J. Fyfe del. W. Archibald

Explanation of Table II.

THE Figures of this Table repreſent, in the Ape and different orders of Quadrupeds, remarkable Varieties of the Size and Shape of the Cavity of the Tympanum; and of its Communication with a Cavern, or with Caverns, analogous to thoſe of our Maſtoid Proceſs.

FIG. 1.

Repreſents the Under Part of the Bones of the Head in the Ape.

A A Protuberance in the Under Part of the Left Os Petroſum.

B A ſimilar Protuberance of the Right Os Petroſum cut, to ſhew a number of Cells, without Marrow, which it contains, and which communicate with the Cavity of the Tympanum.

C A Probe paſſed from the Meatus Auditorius into the Cavity of the Tympanum.

D A Probe paſſed through the Euſtachian Tube into the Cavity of the Tympanum.

Theſe Protuberances, therefore, reſemble in office our Maſtoid Proceſſes, but are differently ſituated.

Fig. 2. reprefents fimilar Protuberances in the Tiger, and Fig. 3. fuch Protuberances in the Sheep: But, on cutting them, Large Caverns, communicating with the Cavity of the Tympanum, are found, inftead of numerous minute Cells.

In the Dog and the Horfe thefe Protuberances agree fo much, in fituation and ftructure, with thofe of the Tiger and Sheep, that I thought it unneceffary to have the Drawings of them Engraved.

It may be worth while to obferve, that, in the Ape, thefe Protuberances are fituated as in the Quadruped; but, that their cellular ftructure correfponds with that of the Human Maftoid Proceffes.

Explanation of Table III.

In this Table, the Offeous Structure of the Human Cochlea and Veftible is reprefented.

FIG. 1.

This Figure fhews, on the Left Side of the Body, the Paffages for the Branches of the Portio Mollis into the Cochlea and Veftible; and the Cavity of the Veftible laid open, on its Backpart, by cutting away a Portion of the Inner and Pofterior Part of the Os Petrofum.

* The

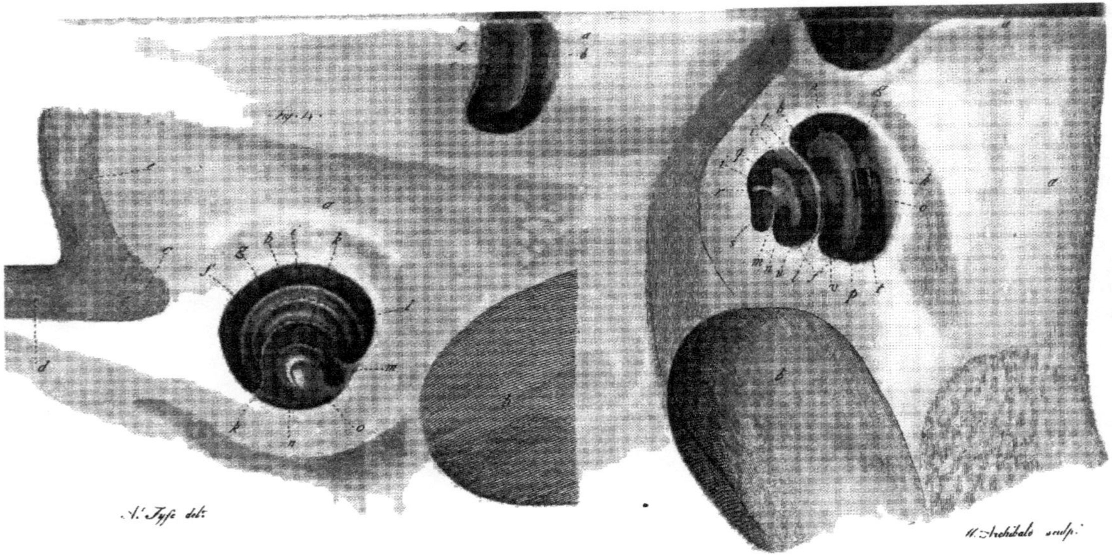

A. Fyfe del.

W. Archibald sculp.

TAB. III.

Fig. 1.

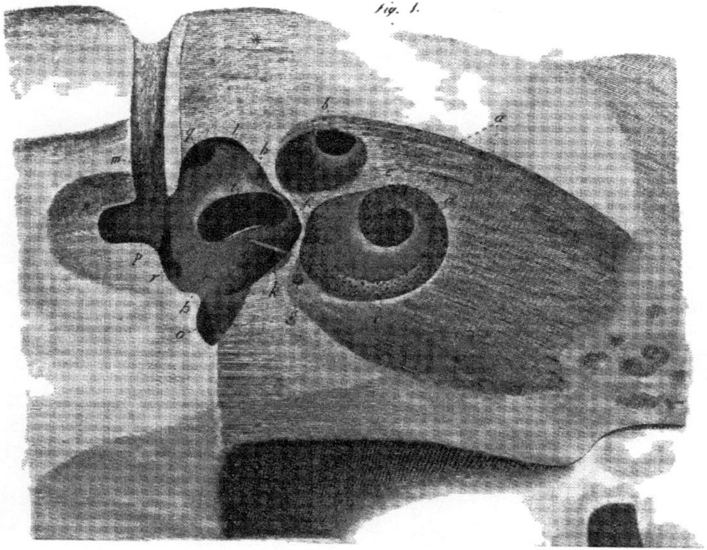

Fig. 2.

* The Inner and Poſterior Part of the Os Petroſum.

a The Bottom of the Canal which contains the Left Branches of the Auditory Nerves.

b The Canal of the Portio Dura of the 7th Pair.

c d A Cribriform Plate, through which the Branches of the Portio Mollis paſs into the Cochlea.

e The Continuation of the ſame Cribriform Plate, forming the Centre and Bottom of the Cavity of the Modiolus.

f g Cribriform Plates, through which Branches of the Portio Mollis paſs into the Veſtible.

h h The Cavity of the Veſtible laid open, by cutting away the Bone which covers its Poſterior Part.

i The Foramen Ovale.

k A Probe paſſed from the Veſtible, into the Scala Veſtibuli of the Cochlea.

l The Anterior, and *m* the Poſterior, End of the Superior Semicircular Canal.

n The Upper, and *o* the Lower, End of the Poſterior Semicircular Canal.

p The Termination, in the Veſtible, of the Tube which is common to the Superior and Poſterior Semicircular Canals, or which is formed by the joining together of their Ends *m n*.

q The Fore, and *r* the Poſterior, End of the Exterior Horizontal Semicircular Canal.

F I G. 2.

Gives a View, from above, of the Cochlea, and Part of the Veſtible and Semicircular Canals, of the Right Side, after cutting away Part of the Os Petroſum.

a The Os Petroſum.

b The Canal for the Internal Carotid Artery.

c The Anterior End of the External Horizontal Semicircular Canal.

d The Anterior End of the Superior Semicircular Canal.

e The Upper Part of the Veſtible.

f The Side of the Cochlea viewed ſomewhat obliquely.

g h i i The Outer Part of the Modiolus, which is Cribriform, or pierced with a number of Holes, for the Paſſage of the Branches of the Portio Mollis.

k A Wire paſſed between Two Plates or Lamellæ, of which the Modiolus conſiſts, and which are at the greateſt diſtance from each other, and therefore beſt ſeen at its Root.

l l The Oſſeous Septum between the Firſt and Second Gyrus of the Cochlea, compoſed of Two Tables or Plates.

m The Oſſeous Septum which ſeparates the Second Gyrus of the Cochlea from the Infundibulum.

n o p The

n o p The First Turn of the Osseous Part or Root of the Lamina Spiralis. At *o* it is cut, to shew that it consists of Two Tables, between which Branches of the Portio Mollis are lodged, which, after dividing into very minute Filaments, pass through innumerable Holes, which are delineated on the Outer Edge of the Osseous Part of the Lamina Spiralis.

q The Second Turn of the Osseous Part of the Lamina Spiralis.

r The Termination of the Lamina Spiralis in a Hamus or Hamulus, the Concave Side of which is connected with, or continued from, the Osseous Septum *m*, which divides the Second Gyrus from the Infundibulum.

s The Infundibulum, at the Bottom of which a Cribriform Osseous Plate is seen, between it and the Apex of the Modiolus, through which Nerves pass from the Modiolus into the Infundibulum.

t u The First and Second Scala of the Tympanum.

v w The First and Second Scala of the Vestible.

FIG. 3.

In this Figure, the Side of the Cochlea is turned a little more outwards than in Fig. 2. by which the Outer Edge of the Lamina Spiralis, and Structure of the Osseous Septum between the Scalæ of the Cochlea, are better seen.

a Represents

a Reprefents the Bafis of the Cochlea.

b The Root of the Cribriform Modiolus.

c The Root of the Lamina Spiralis, which is likewife Cribriform.

d The Outer Edge of the Offeous Part of the Lamina Spiralis, where the Two Laminæ which compofe it are feen, with innumerable Holes for the Paffage of the Branches of the Nerves which are placed between the Laminæ.

e A Section of the Offeous Septum, which divides the Firft from the Second Gyrus of the Cochlea, and which confifts of Two Laminæ.

f The Scala Tympani, and *g* the Scala Veftibuli.

FIG. 4.

Reprefents the Cochlea, and a fmall part of the Semicircular Canals, after cutting off from them the Fore and Outer Part of the Os Petrofum.

a The Fore and Outer Side of the Os Petrofum.

b The Paffage for the Internal Carotid Artery.

c Part of the Veftible.

d The Anterior End of the External Horizontal Semicircular Canal.

e The Anterior End of the Superior Semicircular Canal.

f The Bafis of the Cochlea.

g The Scala of the Tympanum.

h The

TAB. IV.

Fig. 2.

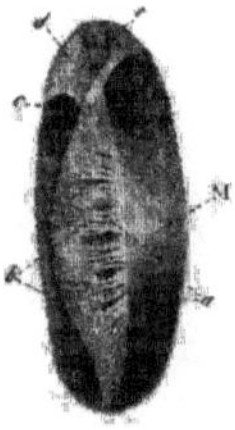

Fig. 3.

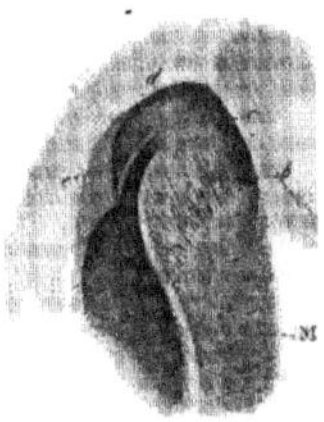

Fig. 1.

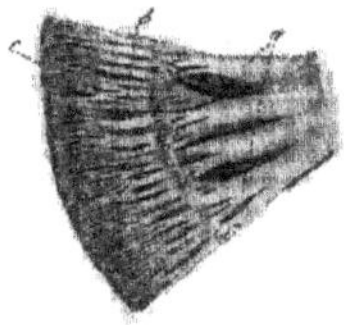

A. Jyss del.

[illegible]

b The Outer Edge of the Oſſeous Part of the Lamina Spiralis, in which there are innumerable Small Holes for the Paſſage of Nerves.

i A Ridge in the Middle of the Oſſeous Part of the Lamina Spiralis, where the Two Plates which compoſe it are at ſuch diſtance from each other as to produce a Riſing or Ridge.

k k The Oſſeous Septum which divides the Firſt from the Second Gyrus of the Cochlea.

l The Scala of the Veſtible.

m The Second Gyrus of the Cochlea.

n The Lamina Spiralis, terminating in a Hamus or Hook.

o The Infundibulum.

Explanation of Table IV.

THE Three Figures of this Table repreſent the Diſtribution of the Branches of the Portio Mollis within the Two Scalæ of the Cochlea, or the Nervous Webs or Retinæ theſe form.

FIG. 1.

Repreſents the Diſtribution of the Branches of the Portio Mollis, on one ſide of the Lamina Spiralis.

a The Large Branches of the Portio Mollis, at the Root or Oſſeous Part of the Lamina Spiralis.

b The

b The Continuation of theſe Branches on the Soft Part of the Lamina Spiralis.

c The Outer Part of the Lamina Spiralis, ſeparated from the Bone of the Cochlea.

Theſe Nerves, in their whole courſe, form an intricate and beautiful Plexus, by repeatedly joining into Trunks, and theſe ſeparating into Branches.

FIG. 2.

M Repreſents the Modiolus.

a The Plexus of Nerves on the Oſſeous Part of the Lamina Spiralis.

b The Plexus of Nerves on the Outer and Softer Part of the Lamina Spiralis.

c The Outer Part of the Lamina Spiralis, dividing into its two conſtituent Layers or Membranes, one of which *d*, continued, lines the Scala of the Veſtible, and the other Layer *e*, continued, lines the Scala of the Tympanum.

FIG. 3.

M Repreſents the Modiolus.

b The Plexus of Nerves on the Lamina Spiralis.

At *c*, the Layer of the Lamina Spiralis, the Continuation of which formed the Retina of the Scala of the Tympanum, is cut off.

d Shews

TAB. V.

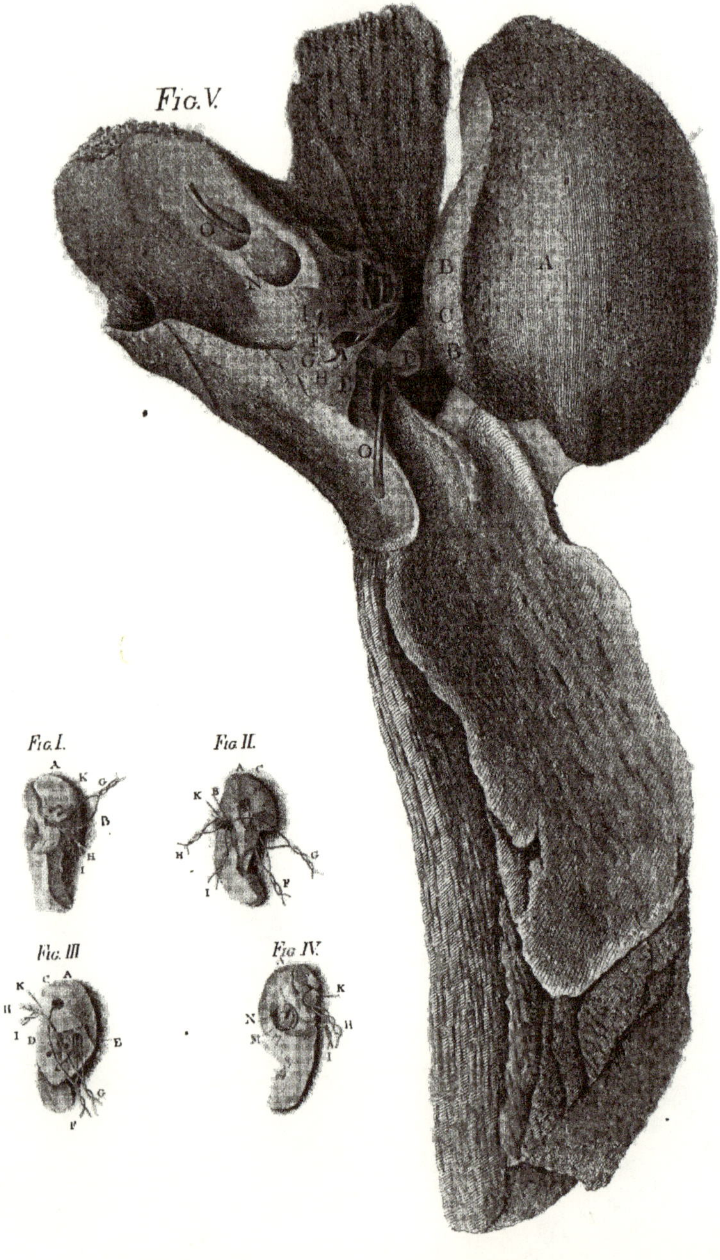

TAB IV.

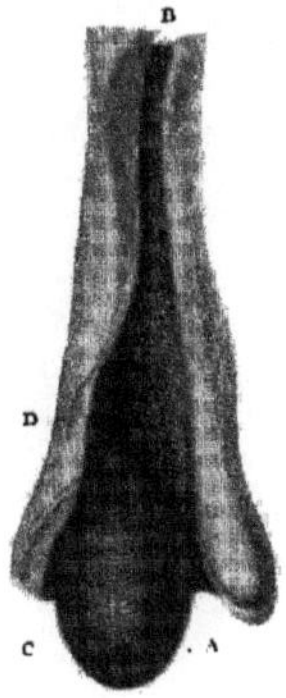

A. [illegible] del.   M. [illegible] Sc.

d Shews the Continuation of the other Layer of the Lamina Spiralis lining the Scala of the Veſtible.

e Is an Inciſion, where the Retina of the Scala Veſtibuli begins to be continued from the Lamina Spiralis.

Explanation of Table IV. *

THIS Table repreſents, of its Natural Size, a Portion of the External Meatus Auditorius of the Cete Balæna, 1. of LINNEUS, laid open.

A The Outer and Wider End of the Meatus.

B The Inner and Narrower Part of it.

C A Smooth Spheroidal Body, the Inner End, or Root, of which, D, is Smaller than its Outer End, and is attached to the Side of the Meatus.

Explanation of Table V.

THE Firſt, Second, Third and Fourth Figures of this Table, repreſent the Veſtible, Semicircular Canals, and Cochlea, of the Cete Delphinus Phocæna of LINNEUS, or of the common Porpoiſe.

The Diameter of all the Parts, which belonged to the Right Ear, is magnified a little; nearly, in proportion to the real Diameter, as Three to Two.

The Same Parts are pointed out by the Same Letters in all the Four Figures.

A The Outer-ſide of the Os Petroſum.

B The Veſtible laid open.

C The Foramen Rotundum.

D E (Fig. 3.) The Apex and Baſis of the Cochlea opened.

F The Ends of a Wire twiſted together, after paſſing it, from the Foramen Rotundum, out at an Opening made into the Scala Tympani of the Cochlea.

G The Ends of a Wire twiſted together, after paſſing it, from the Foramen Ovale, out at an Opening made into the Scala Veſtibuli of the Cochlea.

H The Ends of a Wire twiſted together, after paſſing one end of it, from a Hole in the Superior or Anterior Semicircular Canal, into the Veſtible, and, from that, out at the Foramen Ovale.

I The Ends of a Wire twiſted together, after paſſing both ends of it, from the Cavity of the Poſterior Semicircular Canal, into the Veſtible, and then out at the Foramen Ovale.

These Two Wires are contiguous in the Canal common to the Two Perpendicular Semicircular Canals.

K A Short Wire put into one end of the Third or Horizontal Semicircular Canal.

L The Hole, on the Backpart of the Os Petroſum, for the Paſſage of the Portio Mollis, and Portio Dura of the 7th Pair of Nerves.

M That

M That Branch of the Portio Mollis, which furniſhed Nerves to the Cochlea, dried.

N The other Branch of the Portio Mollis dried, which furniſhed Nerves to the Veſtible and Semicircular Canals.

F I G. 5.

This Figure repreſents the Os Petroſum and the Parts of the Ear, of their Natural Size, in the Cete Phyſeter Macrocephalus of LINNEUS, or the Spermaceti Whale.

A A Part of the Os Petroſum, within which there is a Large Cavity, that communicates with, or makes part of, the Cavity of the Tympanum B B. This is, in Structure and Office, analogous to the Human Maſtoid Proceſs, or to the Hollow Part of the Os Temporum of the Ape and Quadrupeds repreſented in Table II.

C D E The Malleus, Incus, and Stapes, connected to each other by Ligaments. The Root of the Stapes fills the Foramen Ovale.

F A Hole cut in the Bone, in order to ſhew the Cavity of the Veſtible.

G H Two of the Semicircular Canals, cut open to their Terminations in the Veſtible.

I The Scala of the Cochlea which begins at the Foramen Rotundum, which is called Scala Tympani.

K A Probe in the Scala Veſtibuli.

L The Firſt Gyrus of the Cochlea cut open, in which the Oſſeous Root of the Lamina Spiralis is obſervable.

M The Second Gyrus of the Cochlea.

N The Hole which tranſmitted the Portio Mollis of the 7th Pair of Nerves.

O O A Probe in the Winding Canal, which tranſmitted the Portio Dura of the 7th Pair.

Explanation of Table VI.

In this Table, ſome of the Principal Parts of the Ear in the Cete Delphinus Delphis are repreſented.

F I G. 1.

Shews the Orifice of the Meatus Auditorius Externus.

A The Left Eye.

B The Corner of the Mouth.

C D White Lines or Streaks on the ſide of the Head and Body.

E A Briſtle introduced into the Orifice of the Meatus Auditorius Externus.

F I G. 2.

Repreſents the Meatus Auditorius Externus laid open, the Euſtachian Tube and Cavities reſembling thoſe in the Maſtoid

TAB. VI.

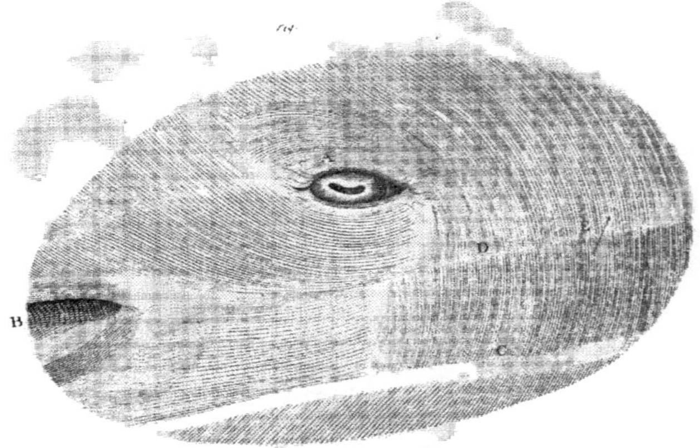

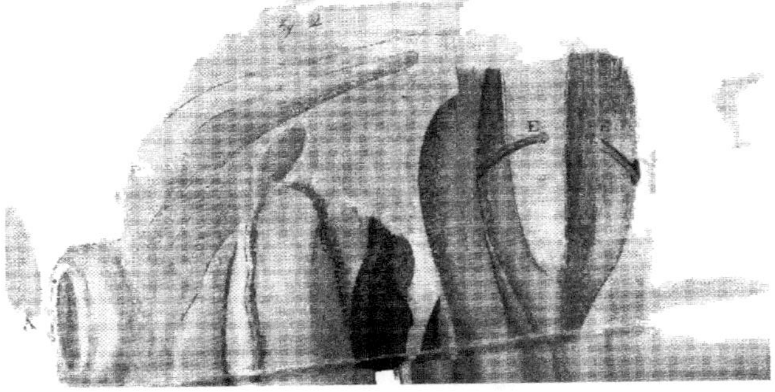

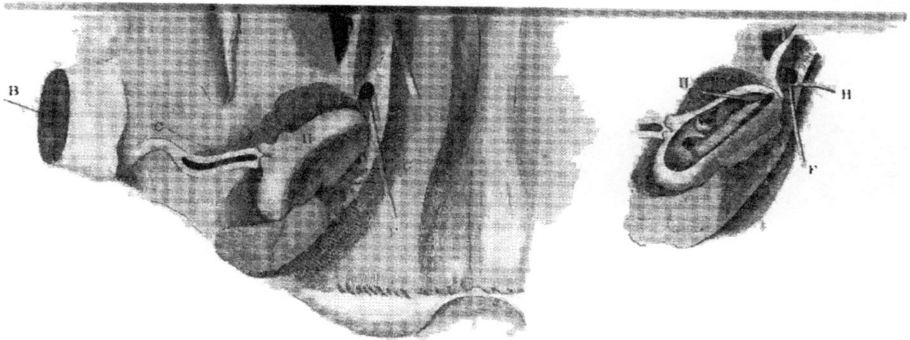

Fig. IV

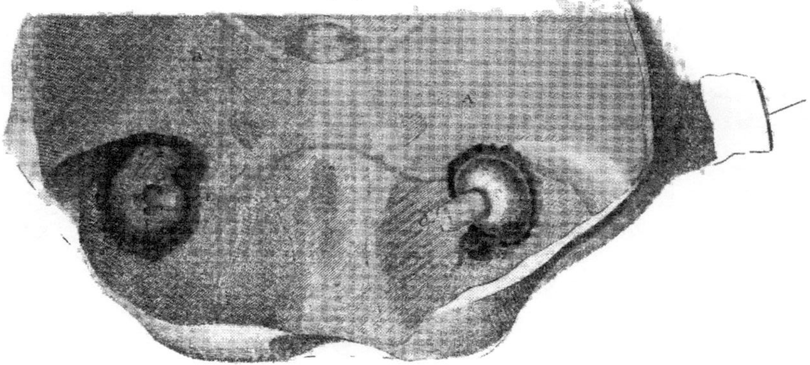

ſtoid Proceſs, with which this Tube and the Cavity of the Tympanum communicate.

A The Eye.

B The Orifice of the Meatus Auditorius with a Briſtle introduced into it.

C The Meatus Auditorius laid open.

E E Probes introduced into the Euſtachian Tubes.

F G The Outer End of the Tube opening into Large Cells.

H A Bone which is Hollow.

In FIG. 3.

F Repreſents the Outer End of the Euſtachian Tube, with a Probe paſſed from it into Large Cells.

Another Probe paſſed from the Outer End of the Euſtachian Tube into the Cavity of the Bone H, the Lower Part of which is cut off, in order to ſhew its Cavity.

FIG. 4.

Shews the Portio Mollis terminating in the Cochlea and Semicircular Canal.

A B The Inner Sides of the Baſe of the Cranium.

C The Trunk of the Portio Mollis.

D The Os Petroſum.

E The Portio Mollis going into the Modiolus.

F G The Sides of the Cochlea laid open.

H One

H One of the Semicircular Canals laid open.

I The Portio Dura of the 7th Pair.

Explanation of Table VII.

The Figures in this Table reprefent the Situation and Connexion of the feveral Canals of the Ear in a Skate Fifh, of their Natural Size.

F I G. 1.

In this Figure, the Situation of the Two Eyes, and of Two Paffages which lead from the Upper Part of the Head into the Throat, and of the feveral Parts of the Brain and Nerves rifing from it, are reprefented, along with the Parts of the Ear.

AAAA Reprefents a Section of the Skin and other Parts of the Upper Side of the Head and Spine.

B B The Eyes.

C C Two Paffages leading down into the Throat.

D The Forepart of the Cavity of the Cranium, which contains fome Cellular Subftance, and is filled with a tranfparent vifcid falt Liquor.

E The Brain.

F The Cerebellum.

1 1 The Olfactory Nerves.

2 2 The Optic Nerves.

33 44 Nerves which refemble the 3d and 4th Pairs.

5 5 Nerves

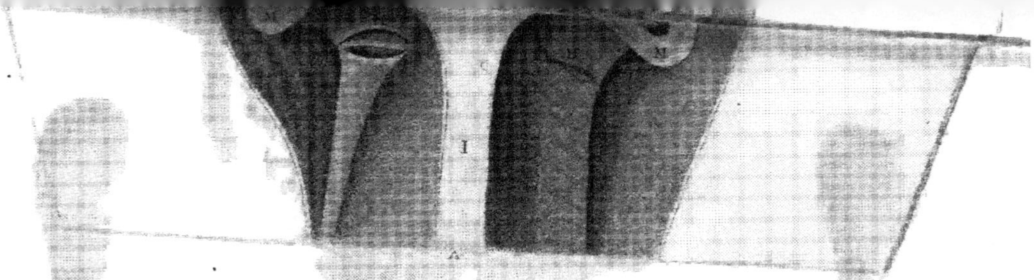

Fig III

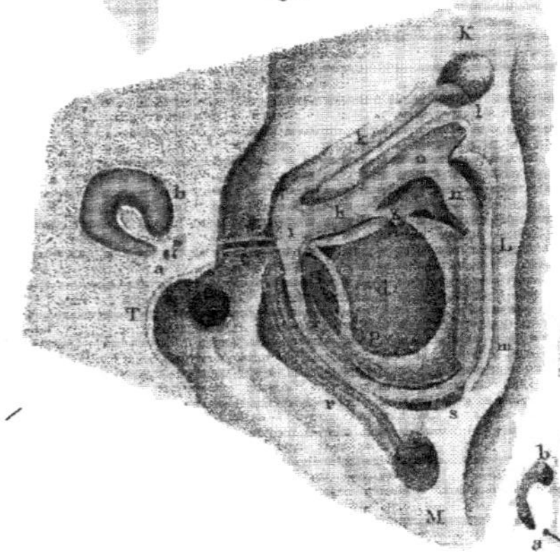

Fig IV

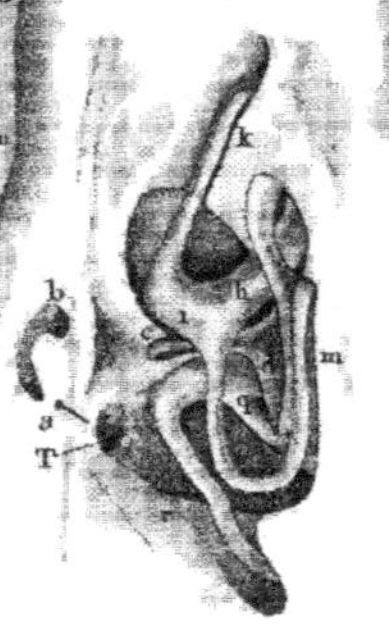

Fig II

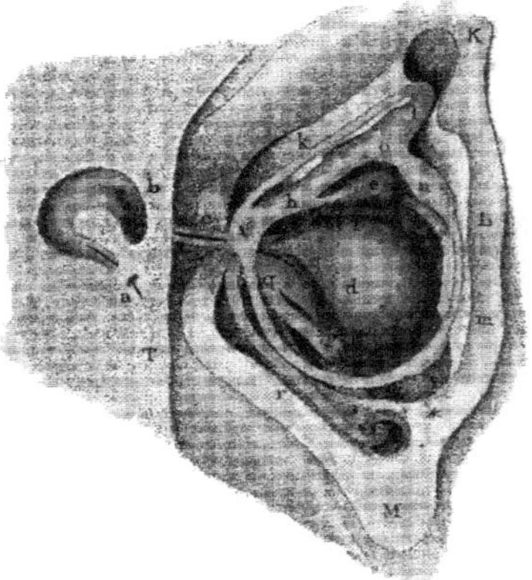

A Fyfe del

Tab. VII.

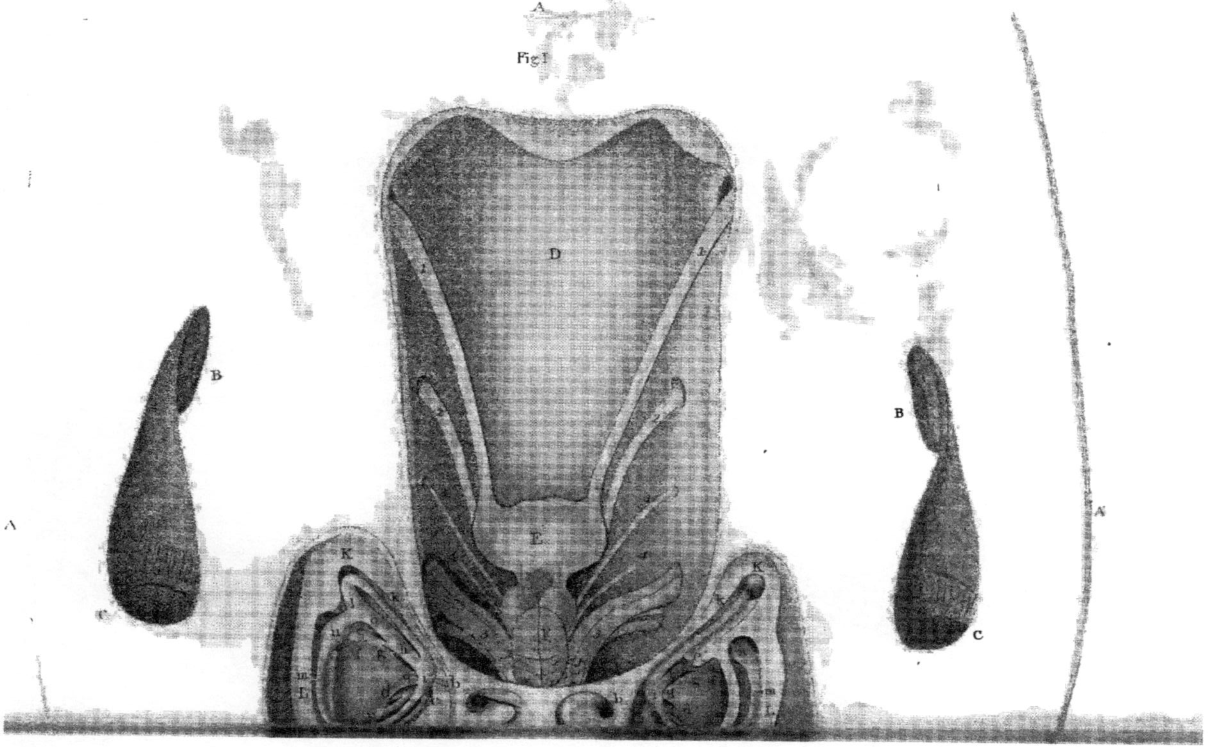

5 5 Nerves which reſemble our 5th Pair, and likewiſe the *Molles* of our 7th Pair.

G The Skin covering the Occiput.

H H The Joints of the Head with the Spine, or Joining of the Condyles of the Occiput with the Firſt Vertebra or Atlas.

I The Skin covering the Spinal Proceſſes of the Vertebræ.

KLM KLM Thick Cartilages, cut horizontally, which cover and contain Three Semicircular, or rather Circular, Canals of the Ear, and certain Sacs, analogous to our Veſtible, with which theſe communicate.

a a The Mouths or Openings of the Meatus Auditorii Externi.

ab ab Winding Canals cut open, which reſemble the Conchæ of the Human Ears.

c A Briſtle paſſed from the Concha of the Left External Ear, into a ſtraight Meatus Auditorius Externus, and, from it, into the Cavity of a Large Sac *d*, reſembling our Veſtible, which is filled, partly with a regularly-ſhaped white ſoft cretaceous Subſtance, and partly with a tranſparent viſcid Fluid.

d In the Right Ear, repreſents the ſame Sac.

e A Small Sac, ſituated on the Forepart of the Large Sac *d*, containing likewiſe a Cretaceous Subſtance and Viſcid Fluid.

* A

* A ſtill Smaller Sac, or rather a Projection from the Backpart of the Large Sac *d*, which alſo contains Cretaceous Matter.

f The Place at which the Large Sac *d* communicates with the Small Sac *e*.

g A Tube leading from the Small Sac *e*, to *h*, which is a Canal common to the Anterior Perpendicular Circular Canal *i k l*, and to the Middle Horizontal Circular Canal *i m n*.

l Is a dilated Part or Bulb in the Anterior Circular Canal, and *n* is a ſimilar Bulb in the Horizontal Circular Canal.

i h o A Large Canal common to the Anterior and Horizontal Middle Canal.

p q A Canal leading from the Inner and Poſterior Part of the Great Sac *d*, to the Poſterior Perpendicular Circular Canal *q r ſ*. At *ſ* there is a Bulb in this Canal, and at its Inferior End *q* it is Wider than it is in its Upper Part.

FIG. 2, 3, 4.

Much Larger Fiſhes than the former were procured for the Preparations repreſented by theſe Three Figures; and in the Preparations repreſented by Fig. 2, 3. the Meatus Auditorius Externus, Veſtible, and the Circular Canals, were injected with

with melted Wax, tinged with three different colours, fuch as thofe with which thefe Figures are painted.

In the Preparation reprefented by Fig. 2. the Veftible was laid in view and delineated, before the injection was thrown in; and the Boundary of the Cretaceous Subftance is feen at the letter *d*.

After all the Canals were injected, in the Preparation reprefented by Fig. 3. the Veftible was cut, and the Wax taken out of it, that its Communications with the Meatus Auditorius Externus, the Small Anterior Sac, and the Canal which leads to the Pofterior Circular Canal, might be more fully feen and delineated.

The feveral Parts reprefented in thefe Three Figures are pointed out by the fame letters as in Fig. 1.; fo that the Explanation already given of Fig. 1. beginning with the letters K L M, applies to Figures 2, 3, 4.

The Meatus Auditorius Externus *c* paffes under the Termination of the Inner-part of the Middle Horizontal Circular Canal, in the Canal *i h o*, common to it and to the Anterior Circular Canal.

Behind the Meatus Auditorius Externus, the Pofterior Circular Canal is contiguous to the Horizontal Circular Canal, but does not communicate directly with it by any Opening.

In Fig. 3. at the letter T, the Outer-fide of a large round Hole or Aperture in the Cartilage which inclofes the Veftible and Circular Canals, is delineated; and, in Fig. 4. at T,

 the

the Inner-ſide of this Hole is repreſented; and, in Fig. 2. at the ſame letter, the Place of the Skin is pointed out, under which this Hole is ſituated.

Explanation of Table VIII.

IN this Table, the Nerves of the Veſtible and Circular Canals in the Right Ear of a Skate are repreſented, after inverting the Head, and cutting away the Cartilages which lie under them.

ABCDE A Section of the Cartilages.

F G The Right Side of the Medulla Oblongata.

H I A Nerve which, in its Diſtribution, reſembles the Human 5th, and Portio Mollis of the 7th Pair.

K A Branch of the Portio Mollis ſent to the Bulb of the Anterior Circular Canal.

L A Branch of it ſent to the Bulb of the Middle Horizontal Circular Canal.

M A Branch of it ſent to the Anterior Sac which communicates with the Veſtible.

N A Number of Branches, forming an elegant Plexus on the under Part of the Veſtible.

O Branches ſent to a Small Projection or Sac at the Under and Poſterior Part of the Veſtible.

P A Branch

TAB. VIII.

Fig. 1.

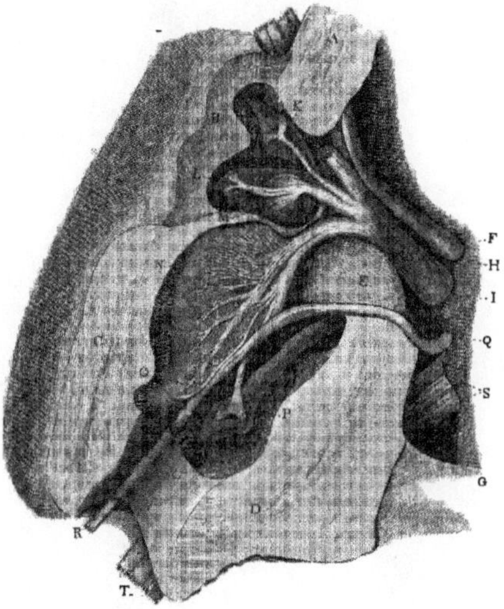

Fig. 3.

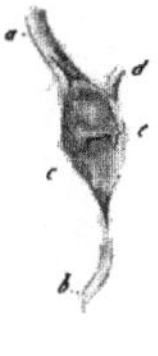

Fig. 2.

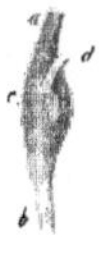

P A Branch ſent to the Bulb of the Poſterior Circular Canal.

Q A Nerve reſembling the Human Portio Dura of the 7th Pair.

S T Nerves reſembling the Human 8th and 9th Pairs of Nerves.

FIG. 2, 3.

Shew, more fully, the way in which the Branches of the Portio Mollis terminate in the Bulbs of the Circular Canals.

a b The Cylindrical Parts of the Circular Canals.

c (Fig. 2.) Shews the Bulb entire; and *c*, in Fig. 3., ſhews the Bulb cut open, in order to bring into view an imperfect Septum, *e*, on which the Nerve ſplits into a great number of minute Branches; which, in a very large Fiſh, weighing upwards of 160 pounds, I have obſerved to form a Plexus on the Septum; and, the Branches then becoming pellucid, it is impoſſible to perceive their farther Diſtribution on the Cylindrical Part of the Circular Canals.

THE END OF TREATISE THIRD.

www.ingramcontent.com/pod-product-compliance
Lightning Source LLC
Chambersburg PA
CBHW021502210326
41599CB00012B/1107
* 9 7 8 3 7 4 1 1 0 4 0 1 5 *